KU-641-834

SOCIAL AND CARING PROFESSIONS IN EUROPEAN WELFARE STATES

Policies, services and professional practices

Edited by Björn Blom, Lars Evertsson and Marek Perlinski

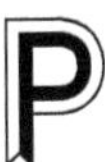

First published in Great Britain in 2017 by

Policy Press
University of Bristol
1-9 Old Park Hill
Bristol
BS2 8BB
UK
t: +44 (0)117 954 5940
pp-info@bristol.ac.uk
www.policypress.co.uk

North America office:
Policy Press
c/o The University of Chicago Press
1427 East 60th Street
Chicago, IL 60637, USA
t: +1 773 702 7700
f: +1 773-702-9756
sales@press.uchicago.edu
www.press.uchicago.edu

British Library Cataloguing in Publication Data
A catalogue record for this book is available from the British Library

Library of Congress Cataloging-in-Publication Data
A catalog record for this book has been requested

ISBN 978-1-4473-2719-6 hardcover
ISBN 978-1-4473-3651-8 ePub
ISBN 978-1-4473-3652-5 Mobi
ISBN 978-1-4473-2721-9 ePdf

Cover design by Policy Press
Front cover image: istock

Contents

List of tables and figures

Notes on contributors

Rasmus Antoft is Dean and Associate Professor of Sociology at the Social Science Faculty, Aalborg University, Denmark. His academic interests include qualitative research methods, the sociology of professions and organisations, creative methods and the sociology of health and illness. His most recent research has focused on organisational change in the healthcare sector, interprofessional relations in healthcare, patient education and the history of the Chicago School of Sociology.

Jim Barry is a political sociologist. He is Professor Emeritus at the University of East London, UK and Visiting Professor at Luleå University of Technology, Sweden. He holds editorial board appointments with *Gender, Work & Organization* and *Equality, Diversity and Inclusion*. His research interests include social work, higher education, gender, management, and the public sector more generally. He has worked collaboratively and published widely with his co-authors for this edited collection, Professor Elisabeth Berg, Professor John Chandler and Dr Marion Ellison. His publications have appeared in a number of books and journals, the latter including *Gender, Workand Organization*, *Human Relations*, *Soziale Welt* and *Organization*.

Liz Beddoe is an Associate Professor in the Faculty of Education and Social Work, University of Auckland, New Zealand. Liz's teaching and research interests include critical perspectives on social work education and professional supervision. Liz has published articles on supervision and professional issues in New Zealand and international journals. Recent books include the co-authored *Challenges in Professional Supervision* (Jessica Kingsley Publishers, 2016) with Allyson Davys, *Social Work Practice for Promoting Health and Wellbeing: Critical Issues* (Routledge, 2014), and *Social Policy for Social Work and Human Services in Aotearoa New Zealand: Diverse Perspectives* (Canterbury University Press, 2016) with Jane Maidment.

Linda Bell is an Associate Professor in the School of Health and Education, Middlesex University, London (United Kingdom). She has researched various aspects of health, social care and family life and has a PhD in anthropology. She has taught social work and other professional students since 1995, with a focus on research methodology and ethics. She has published widely in journals including *Aging and Mental Health, Equal Opportunities International, Journal of Interprofessional*

Care, Social Work Education, Sociological Review and *Women's Studies International Forum*. Her recent books are *Research Methods for Social Workers* (Palgrave MacMillan, in press) and *Ethics, Values and Social Work Practice*, edited with Trish Hafford-Letchfield (Open University Press (McGraw-Hill), 2015).

Elisabeth Berg is Professor in Sociology at the Department of Human Work Sciences, Luleå University of Technology, Sweden and Visiting Professor at the University of East London, United Kingdom. Her research concerns gender, organisation, social politics and management in academia in Sweden and England. She has published a number of books and articles in peer-reviewed journals. Two of her most recent publications exploring evidence-based practice are 'The Uncertain Rise of Evidence-based Practice in Social Work in Sweden and England in Contexts Framed by New Public Management and Neo-liberalism' with J. Barry and J. Chandler, in *Sorge: Arbeit, Verhältnisse* (Nomos Verlagsgesellschaft mbH & Co., 2014) and 'Neoliberalism, managerialism and the reconfiguring of social work in Sweden and the United Kingdom', with E. Harlow, J. Barry and J. Chandler, *Organization*, 20 (4).

Björn Blom is Professor of Social Work at the Department of Social Work, Umeå University, Sweden. His research interests are organisations, professions, knowledge-use, evaluation and addiction treatment. He has taught social work students since 1991, with a focus on the evaluation of social work practice. He has published widely in journals including *Evaluation and Program Planning, Journal of Social Work, Journal of Critical Realism, Professions and Professionalism*. He has co-authored and co-edited seven books on knowledge, organisations, social work practice and evaluation. His recent book (together with Stefan Morén) is *Teori för social arbete* (Studentlitteratur, 2015).

John Chandler is Professor of Work and Organisation at the Royal Docks School of Business and Law, University of East London, United Kingdom. His research interests lie in identity and diversity in the workplace, particularly in the public service context. Publications include *Identity at Work* (Routledge, 2016) and, as co-editor, *Questioning the New Public Management* (Ashgate Publishing, 2004).

Marion Ellison is a Reader in European Social and Public Policy at Queen Margaret University in Edinburgh as well as Visiting Professor in Comparative Welfare States at Ca'Foscari University in

Venice, Italy. Specialising and publishing widely in comparative social policy, social work, public management, governance and work and employment in Europe, she has collaborated extensively with her co-authors Professor Elisabeth Berg, Professor Jim Barry and Professor John Chandler. As permanent partner for Scotland for the EU (FP7) INSPIRES Project (Innovative Social Policies for Inclusive and Resilient Labour Markets in Europe), Marion authored the final report to the European Commission informing EU 2020 recommendations, as well as the policy briefs for national and local governments across Europe. Her forthcoming book, *Policy Lessons and Innovations for Improving Young People's Transitions into Work* (2017, Edward Elgar), examines the impact, on young people across Europe, of the social and employment policies adopted after the 2008 financial crisis.

Lars Evertsson has a PhD in Sociology from the Department of Sociology, Umeå University, and is Associate Professor of Social Work at the Department of Social Work, Umeå University, Sweden. His research explores the interface between welfare policies, the organisation of welfare services and development of welfare professional groups. As a teacher he has taught on undergraduate, graduate and PhD level courses in social work and sociology. He has been published in journals and books in Swedish and English.

Krystyna Faliszek has a PhD in Sociology from the University of Silesia, and is Associate Professor at the Institute of Sociology, University of Silesia. She took part in a research project that explored educational needs in social work and the use of local social policy to solve social problems. She was the leader of a project on tackling social problems in Katowice. The project was financed with EU funds and was a collaboration between the University of Silesia and the local government of Katowice. She is the president of the examination board for social workers, which operates from the office of the governor of Silesia. Her main research interests include social policy, social work, social problems and social exclusion.

Anders Hanberger is Professor in Evaluation at Umeå University, Sweden. He has published articles on evaluation of public policies and programmes, evaluation systems, the interplay of evaluation and governance, and evaluation methodology. He has a particular interest in the role of evaluation in democracy and accountability, and the consequences and constitutive effects of evaluation.

Kåre Heggen is Professor of Social Science at the Faculty of Social Science and History, Volda University College, Norway, and also at the Centre of the Study of Professions (CSP), Oslo og Akershus University College, Norway. His main research area is education and educational sociology, especially the education and qualification of professionals from universities and colleges (teachers, social workers and nurses). He has published books and articles in these areas.

Kjeld Høgsbro is Professor of Social Work at Aalborg University, Denmark. He has published books on disabilities, mental illness, social work and community development in Denmark. As Senior Research Fellow at The Danish Institute of Governmental Research he conducted evaluations of programmes for substance abuse and homelessness, as well as for people with mental illness, brain injuries and pervasive developmental disorders. He has developed models for coherent services for young people with physical disabilities, models for community psychiatry in Denmark and models for studying rehabilitation schemes. He has been a board member of research committees on the sociology of mental health and sociological practice at The International Sociological Association.

Joakim Isaksson is a Senior Lecturer and Researcher in Social Work at Umeå University, Sweden. His research interests include the organisation of psychosocial resources in school and in cancer care. He has previously published in the area of special needs in the education system. Currently he is focused on exploring how patients with head and neck cancer resume everyday life after treatment, as well as the implications on the organisation of rehabilitation for these patients, and the function of the social worker in cancer care and rehabilitation.

Ilse Julkunen is Professor in Practice Research at the Department of Social Research, University of Helsinki, Finland. Her research concerns youth unemployment and marginalisation, youth transitions, comparative research and practice research. She is the scientific leader of the practice research milieu of the Mathilda Wrede Institute at the Centre of Excellence of Social Welfare in Helsinki. She is a social worker and has worked at the Institute of Welfare and Health. Together with Edgar Marthinsen she has co-edited *Practice Research in Nordic Social Work: Knowledge production in transition* (Whiting and Birch, 2012). Recently she has co-edited, with Gillian Ruch, *Relationship-based Research in Social Work* (Jessica Kingsley Publishers, 2016).

Hildur Kalman is Professor of Social Work and Associate Professor in the Philosophy of Science and RPT at the Department of Social Work, Umeå University, Sweden. Her main research interests are methodology, ethics and emotions. Recent publications focus on the challenges of intimate care in home care services, and field education for social work students.

Synnöve Karvinen-Niinikoski is Professor (Emerita) of Social Work in the Faculty of Social Sciences, University of Helsinki, Finland. Her research and teaching interests have included critical reflection, professional supervision and reflective structures, transformative professional agency and expertise, social work practice research and international social work research. She has been active in the Nordic and international development of social work education and research and is a member of the IASSW Research Committee. Her international publications include 'How can we enhance productivity in social work? Dynamically reflective structures and dialogic leadership for transformative expertise' (*Journal of Social Work Practice*, 2013/2, jointly with Laura Yliruka) and a special issue on practice research for the *Nordic Journal of Social Work Research* (2014, edited jointly with Ilse Julkunen).

Lena Lindgren is Associate Professor in Public Administration at Gothenburg University, Sweden. She works with teaching and research focusing on the theory and practice of evaluation and policy analysis. Her current research explores the implications of a crowded policy space: how policies and evaluation systems in the field of education interfere with each other in ways that have unintended consequences.

Witold Mandrysz has an MA in Sociology and a PhD in Sociology, both from the University of Silesia, Poland. He is a teacher and researcher in the Social Work Unit at the Institute of Sociology, University of Silesia. He is also involved in several international, national and regional research projects. His main research interests are social work, social economy, community work, participation and civic dialogue, and local governance.

Maria Appel Nissen is Associate Professor in Social Work at Aalborg University, Denmark. Since the mid-1990s she has been engaged in the development of social work, in particular social work with families and children. Her research focuses on the practices and forms of knowledge in social work, and how they relate to: knowledge in science; social problems (as well as how we perceive them); and wider structural, political and organisational changes within society. Currently she is heading a research project titled 'Views on Human Beings in Social Work – Welfare Policies, Technologies and Knowledge about human beings' (2014–2017). She is the editor of *Nordic Social Work Research*.

Urban Nothdurfter is Assistant Professor of Social Work at the Free University of Bozen, Italy. He is a qualified social worker and holds a PhD in sociology and social research from the University of Trento, Italy. His research interests focus on the relations between social policy development and social work practice, particularly the street-level delivery of activation policies, social work history and professionalisation, and on LGBTQ issues in social work.

Lennart Nygren is Professor of Social Work at Umeå University, Sweden. He has authored or edited books on auditing, evaluation, social policy and social work. He has published research papers in different sub-fields of social work, for example child protection, family-based interventions, youth health, and qualitative and comparative methodology.

Søren Peter Olesen is Associate Professor in Social Work at Aalborg University, Denmark. His research explores employment-oriented social work and user perspectives on the consequences of social work in this field. He belongs to a research group exploring social work at the street-level of employment policy implementation. This group is based at the Department of Sociology and Social Work, Aalborg University. Recently he has been involved in two major mixed-methods projects on jobcentre-workers and on progression in work readiness among vulnerable unemployed citizens.

Sabina Pawlas-Czyz is a Lecturer at the Institute of Sociology at University of Silesia, Poland. She holds a PhD in Sociology and is a psychologist. She has been devoted to training future social workers for 18 years and created and organised the second degree specialisation of social work at the University of Silesia. In her research, she focuses on social work with chosen groups of clients, as well as the sociology of health and disease (especially oncological and terminal), the sociology of families in crisis situations (situations of loss), and the education and professional improvement of professional social services.

Marek Perlinski is a Senior Lecturer in Social Work at the Department of Social Work, Umeå University, Sweden. His research interests include professional and organisational aspects of public service social services. He has degrees in sociology and personnel administration (HR). He has extensive experience of academic teaching in sociology (since 1986) and social work (since 1999). He contributed to a number of textbooks in social work and also published in international scientific journals such as the *Journal of Social Work*, *Social Work & Society* and *Administration in Social Work* and some Nordic scientific journals.

Devin Rexvid has a PhD in social work from the Department of Social Work, Umeå University, Sweden. In his research he compares social workers' and general practitioners' enactment of practice in relation to the Swedish government's efforts on knowledge governance of these professions' practice. Devin Rexvid also has research interests in, and publications on, masculinity and honour-related violence.

Gillian Ruch is Professor of Social Work and Head of the Department of Social Work and Social Care at the University of Sussex. She teaches and researches in the areas of child care social work and relationship-based and reflective practice and is committed to enhancing the wellbeing of children, families and practitioners. Her particular interests are in promoting psycho-social research methods and reflective forums that facilitate relationship-based practice. Gillian's current research includes an ESRC funded four UK nations project exploring how social workers communicate with children, and an ESRC Knowledge Exchange Project introducing a cognitive and affective supervisory model to child and family social workers. Gillian has co-edited, with Danielle Turney and Adrian Ward, *Relationship-based Social Work: Getting to the Heart of Practice* (Jessica Kingsley Publishers, 2010) and her recent publication *Relationship-Based Research in Social Work: Understanding Practice Research* (Jessica Kingsley Publishers, 2016), is co-edited with Ilse Julkunen from the University of Helsinki.

Lars Inge Terum is a Professor at the Centre for the Study of Professions (CSP), Oslo and Akershus University College, Norway. He was educated as a social worker in 1974 and in 1996 he received a PhD in Sociology from the University of Oslo, Norway. His research explores the implementation of public policy, discretionary decision-making and professional competence. He was the founder director of CSP and has been coordinator of the PhD programme in the Study of Professions.

Eline Thornquist is Professor of Physiotherapy at Bergen University College, Norway and at University of Tromsø, The Norwegian Arctic University. She has published widely in national and international journals and has written several books. Her main research interests are practice in natural settings, text analyses, and the theory of science.

Daniel Törnqvist holds a PhD in Sociology, and is currently working as a Senior Lecturer in the Department of Social Work, Umeå University, Sweden. His research interest concerns addiction, primarily on a policy level. His dissertation focused on the debate over narcotics in Sweden between the years 1970–1999. He also focuses on training future social workers, mainly in courses on scientific method.

Ming-sum TSUI is Professor of Social Work and Associate Dean at the Faculty of Health & Social Sciences, The Hong Kong Polytechnic University, Hong Kong. He received his MSW from McGill University and earned his PhD from the University of Toronto. His research interests include social work supervision, human service management, the theory and practice of social work, social work education and substance abuse. He has published more than 130 items of research, including *Social Work Supervision: Contexts and Concepts* (Sage, 2005) and 60 refereed journal articles.

Jorunn Vindegg is an Associate Professor at Oslo and Akershus University College of Applied Sciences, Norway. Her research interests include knowledge for practice – the knowledge foundation for social work and child welfare – as well as practice-based research and research-based practice within social work and child welfare. She was the editor of *The Journal of Norwegian Child Welfare* for 12 years, and is currently head of the Ethical Committee of the Norwegian Union of Social Educators and Social Workers.

Elisabeth Willumsen is a Professor in Social Work at the University of Stavanger, Norway. She was educated as a social worker, has a masters in special education and a PhD in public health from the Nordic School of Public Health, Gothenburg, titled 'Interprofessional collaboration in residential childcare'. Her research and publications have focused on interprofessional collaboration/collaborative work and service-user participation in welfare contexts, particularly child welfare, and additionally between academia and practice (practice research). Recently, the area of social innovation in the public sector has become central to her research projects, which have received funding from the EU and the Norwegian Research Council. Willumsen holds a Professor II position at Molde University College and a co-position at the Centre of Innovation Research (UiS), Molde, Norway.

Kazimiera Wódz is Professor of Sociology and Head of the Social Work Unit at the Institute of Sociology, Faculty of Social Sciences, University of Silesia, Poland. She created the social work educational programme at the Faculty (BA studies and MA studies). Kazimiera is a member of the editorial board of *Social Work & Society*, *Social Space* and is an editor of the series *Problems of Social Work* (published by Akapit Publishing House in Toruń). She was chair of the social work division of the Polish Sociological Association from 2009 to 2015. Her academic work explores the revitalisation of squalid town districts, the activation of communities threatened by social exclusion, the professionalisation of social work in Poland, and the development of civic dialogue and public participation at local levels.

Preface

In most countries in Europe, and in several other parts of the world, almost everyone has contact with social and caring welfare professionals at different stages of life. For example, most people have recurrent contact with physicians, but many also have contact with social workers or other social and caring professionals within in a social security system. It is fairly safe to say that such welfare professions in recent decades have become increasingly important for individuals as well as whole societies. Previous research on welfare professions has to a great extent focused on certain professional groups or professions in a specific country. This book intends to offer broader knowledge by presenting research-based knowledge on various aspects of social and caring welfare professions from a European perspective. It also wishes to offer detailed insights into welfare professionals' daily work with clients and patients.

The Network for Comparative Research on Professions (N-CORP) was founded in spring 2010. It consists of researchers within the social sciences and medicine in a number of European countries. The network aims to contribute to the theoretical and empirical research on welfare professions, and to disseminate this knowledge within as well as outside academia. In light of these ambitions, the members of N-CORP decided to write this book.

Since the book is written by members of a network, it is largely the result of teamwork between the participating authors and editors. During several physical and computer-based meetings, we discussed focus and form concerning the book as a whole as well as individual chapters. The design of the book and the review of the content have thus largely been a joint process.

The book consists of four sections. Part 1 focuses on knowledge, reflection and identity in the social and caring welfare professions; Part 2 examines control, regulation and management; Part 3 discusses collaboration, conflict and competition; and Part 4 concentrates on assessment, negotiation and decision making. Taken together, the chapters within these four themes highlight and problematise key aspects of current European social and caring professions.

Whether you will read this book in its entirety, or choose to focus on individual chapters, it is appropriate to acknowledge that the authors are aware that social and caring welfare professions is a broad label for a wide range of occupations that perform a variety of tasks aimed at different groups of people with diverse needs and problems. Moreover, welfare professionals work within a variety of organisations that have differing conditions in different countries. The book therefore does not aim to convey a comprehensive picture of the social and caring welfare professions in Europe. Nor does it intend to say how welfare professionals' work should be conducted. The intention with this book is to discuss and problematise a number of aspects regarding social and caring welfare professions in European welfare states that we regard as particularly central and hitherto little discussed from a European perspective. Overall, we hope that the book will serve as a source of critical reflection, insight and inspiration, both for those who read about social and caring welfare professions in European welfare states for the first time and for those who already have some knowledge in the field.

In addition to the authors representing N-CORP, several researchers from other parts of the world have participated in this effort, numbering in total 34 authors from nine countries. We would like to express our sincere appreciation to all the authors, who spared no effort to contribute to the book. We also want to express our gratitude to Isobel Bainton, commissioning editor at Policy Press, whose positive attitude and practical support during different parts of the process was invaluable.

The primary audiences for this book are students, educators and researchers in social and medical sciences, as well as within humanities. The book is relevant to students and educators since aspects of professionalism and professionalisation are increasingly taught and discussed in higher education, especially in programmes preparing for work within the human services. The book is also relevant to researchers, as interest in professions, professionalism and professionalisation has spread to disciplines than other sociology. These include, for example, theoretical disciplines such as political science and philosophy of science, and especially applied disciplines such as social work, medicine, psychology and physiotherapy.

The secondary audience is practitioners within these disciplines. The book is relevant to practitioners since it puts professional practice in a broader political and cultural context. This can help practitioners to understand how significant political changes across Europe affect welfare policy and shape their everyday practice.

Björn Blom, Lars Evertsson and Marek Perlinski

ONE

European social and caring professions in transition

Björn Blom, Lars Evertsson and Marek Perlinski

Introduction

The European welfare state has existed in institutionalised form since the 1880s, with the gradual launch of the Bismarck system,[1] and in its contemporary form since after the Second World War. However, the William Beveridge report from 1942 is often regarded as having laid the foundation for the welfare state (Quadagno, 1987; Baldwin, 1990; Korpi and Palme, 1998; Kuhnle, 2000: Healy, 2009). A prominent feature of European welfare states is the existence of different professions with the task of implementing the ideals of taking care of its citizens, in particular weak and vulnerable groups. Some professions evolved long before the advent of the welfare state (for example, medicine and nursing), while others emerged in its wake (for example, social work and audiology).

Since the mid-1980s we have witnessed an increasing number of social and caring welfare professions, as more vocational groups have received a higher education. Moreover, vocational education at university level has become increasingly theoretical, and more professionals have received a licence to practise. Such changes can be said to reflect an increased professionalisation and academisation of previously known semi-professional groups (Ek et al, 2013).

In principle, professionalisation has increased the opportunities for handling various societal problems, by creating occupational groups that can use abstract knowledge independently in diverse situations. From a state perspective, this is usually one of the reasons for initiating and supporting professionalisation. At the same time, professionalisation has strengthened various occupational groups in their efforts to develop a stronger professional identity (Adams et al, 2006; Mieg, 2008), to gain recognition, influence and autonomy. This part of the process is not always perceived as positive from a state perspective, not least because autonomous professionals can be more difficult to govern and control.

Recently, however, several welfare professions have experienced an escalation in control and governance by the state, and hence reduced autonomy and professional discretion. Some argue that this constitutes an ongoing deprofessionalisation, whereby welfare professionals will have diminished opportunities to act from professional principles (Guzman, 2012). Others argue, however, that increased governance and control does not affect professionals' work that much, since *discretion* is fundamental in professional practice and cannot be omitted (Jessen, 2011).

Several researchers claim that today's society is permeated by assessment, monitoring, evaluation and inspection, to the extent that we can talk about an audit society. One clear feature of many welfare organisations is that they spend much of their time and energy on auditing. Since welfare professionals nowadays are embedded in organisations, they will be affected in several ways: they will be audited, and will also conduct audits (Power, 1999; Forsell and Ivarsson Westerberg, 2014). Some scholars even argue that the growing phenomenon of supervision can be seen in light of the audit society, since supervision can work both as an instrument for developing professionalism and safeguarding autonomy, as well as a way to impose different forms of governance and monitoring of welfare professionals (Manthorpe et al, 2015).

Another significant trait of modern societies is the increased organisational specialisation – division of functions – that often necessitates collaboration between different groups in order to achieve a holistic view of citizens', often complex, problems (Blom, 2004; Bergmark and Lundström, 2007). By way of example, doctors, social workers and therapists sometimes need to work with the same multi-problem families. But the same conditions that necessitate collaboration can also hamper interaction because there is competition between different professions. Within organisations, conflicts and demarcation problems arise as more professions claim to be the most suited to handle a certain task (Rose, 2011). For example, in the healthcare system several groups claim to be able to offer social support and counselling (medical social workers, nurses, psychologists and so on).

Another source of conflict between professional groups is that there are often different ways of viewing people's problems. For example, several researchers argue that currently there is a medicalisation of social problems where, for example, drug abuse and hyperactivity among children are regarded as medical rather than social problems (Conrad and Potter, 2000; Conrad and Schneider, 2010). Fundamentally it is often a struggle for power and resources that is reflected in so-called domain conflicts, where there is a 'tug of war' between various professional groups.

According to Andrew Abbott's classical model (2014), professional work is divided into three parts: diagnosis, inference and treatment. The basic idea is that professionals use their formal knowledge, in a rather rational and systematic way, in order to understand what a client's problem is, to figure out what to do, and then do something about it. In this scenario, the professional is the most active agent, and the client rather passive. An example could be the contact between a physician and a patient with heart problems. Although Abbott's model to some extent is valid for the welfare professions, there are reasons to question it. One reason is that many welfare professionals deal with problems and conditions that are quite different from those experienced by professionals such as engineers, whose work fits Abbott's model more easily. For example, social workers often stand before abstract psychosocial phenomena (such as honour-related oppression) that are not possible to 'diagnose' from the professional's perspective alone, but can only be understood if the client is actively involved in the process of co-constructing the problem.

Another reason is that welfare professions are affected by an increasing emphasis on users' preferences, participation and influence. The professional has gone from being regarded as an 'expert who knows best', to being seen as someone who is expected to have a more equal relationship with users such as clients and patients. An imaginable consequence of this for professionals is, for example, that it could become more complicated, time-consuming and expensive to provide support, since it is insufficient to start from the professionals' point of view in interactions with service users. Ideally, users should be involved in the entire process of defining problems and making decisions as well as carrying out interventions. This situation is accentuated because today's citizens are more knowledgeable about their rights and the help options available (Kim et al, 2011; Rexvid et al, 2012).

Professional groups have also experienced the effects of economic policy changes in line with increased market orientation, often with increasing privatisation, of the public sector in many countries (Segev et al, 2012). A consequence of this is the introduction of competition, which means that public and private welfare providers compete for resources and work tasks. Another is that financial responsibility is delegated and imposed on individual professionals, implying that they have to weigh the need for interventions in specific cases against its costs and the organisation's budget.

Other challenges that welfare professionals are confronted with follow from increased mobility between countries (Bijak et al, 2013), bringing, for example, new forms of substance abuse and service users with different types of needs that can evoke difficulties regarding ethics and equity (Ellett et al, 2007). A possible consequence is that professionals will not know how to act in certain circumstances due to lack of knowledge about new phenomena that accompany migration. Another consequence is the emergence of ethical uncertainty about how to act in relation to people with different ethnic or religious backgrounds, out of fear of behaving in an offensive manner.

All in all, it is noticeable that welfare professions in Europe have undergone considerable changes during recent decades (Laffin and Entwistle, 2000; Healy, 2009; Beach, 2011). It is clear that many professions are facing new demands and expectations, which represent challenges that are crucial to understand in a more qualified way. Such knowledge is important to professionals themselves, as well as to policymakers, educators and the users of welfare services. The issues discussed here highlight a number of concerns that, raised as four questions, make up the starting point for this book:

- How are social and caring welfare professionals' identities influenced by education, work experience and supervision?
- How are social and caring welfare professions affected by governance, regulation and control by the state?
- How are social and caring welfare professions affected by collaboration, conflict and competition with other welfare professions?
- How do social and caring welfare professionals, in practice, assess and make decisions in their work with clients and patients?

In the following chapters these questions are addressed by authors who, with their different perspectives and experiences, show that the questions are not only important but also difficult to answer.

The aim of the book is to provide new insights about current social and caring welfare professions and their practices in a number of European countries in a comprehensive and structured way. By presenting research-based knowledge, the book intends to offer the following insights:

- An understanding of the current practices of social and caring welfare professions in countries with different cultural, social and political contexts.

- Deeper knowledge about the subtle, dynamic, affective and interactive aspects of professional work. This challenges the view that social and caring welfare professionals' work concentrates on rational use of knowledge.
- An understanding of the contextual factors influencing professionals' work (for example, government control, organisation models and interprofessional collaboration).
- Knowledge concerning the ways in which attitudes, emotions, identities and education affect professional work.

Social and caring welfare professions

The concept 'professions' has varied with different researchers and in different historical periods, but roughly speaking it is possible to discern two different approaches to what a profession is: an essentialist and a procedural approach (Freidson, 2001; Molander and Terum, 2008; Jessen, 2011; Abbott, 2014). The essentialist approach assumes that professions can be defined and described using a number of properties or attributes. This type of definition emanates from Ernest Greenwood (1957) stating that professions seem to have a number of specific characteristics, for example systematic theory, professional authority, societal sanction and ethical rules. However, this essentialist approach has been criticised. An important part of the criticism focuses on the notion of value consensus: the assumption that professionals are altruistic and without self-interest for society and citizens (Freidson, 1970; Johnson, 1972; Safatti-Larson, 1977).

This contrasts with the procedural approach, which emphasises competition and border disputes between occupational groups who want to increase their power and influence. The procedural approach points to significant vested interests: the pursuit of power, influence, higher salary and good working conditions for the members of a profession. In practice this means competition with other professions about so-called jurisdiction, the power and authority to carry out tasks in a particular field (Abbott, 2014).

In a European context the concept 'social and caring welfare professions' has somewhat different meanings in different countries. For example, there are differing levels of integration between health services and social services in different countries. In some countries welfare is more related to social interventions than to medical or health interventions. This book deals with this by defining the concept social and caring welfare profession relatively broadly, as occupational groups with an academic degree (bachelor or higher) that possess a certain amount of institutionalised and somewhat unique knowledge. These groups work within a range of social, caring and healthcare services, provided by public organisations in order to improve or maintain quality of life for individuals and groups. In general, they also have a certain amount of professional autonomy regarding how to carry out work tasks.

Another significant feature of social and caring welfare professions is their close connection to the state. Sometimes the state itself *creates* new professions, for instance social insurance officers, based on perceived welfare-state needs. It is also possible for the state to *incorporate* professions that have emerged independently of any state intervention, for example physicians. Moreover, the state can *transform* occupations into professions, even when it had nothing to do with the creation of the original occupation; for example, the state had no influence over what might be termed 'the original charity workers',[2] but it did have a hand in turning unskilled charity workers into social workers by way of a university education. This transformation has happened at different times in different countries, and has often been a process that stretched over several decades. While some professions, like architects, have emerged and exist without any connection to the state, it is difficult to imagine welfare professions without such a link.

Examples of social and caring welfare professionals embraced in the book are: social workers, physicians, physiotherapists, elderly care workers, psychologists, family assistants, community workers, psychiatrists and job centre officers. There are several motives for including these groups as examples of European social and caring welfare professions: first, these professions exist in several European countries and are hence relatively representative; second, they are quite common, so knowledge concerning them can be generalised to other welfare professions; and third, they represent a spectrum of social and caring welfare professions, which enables a broad understanding of the current situation in European welfare states.

In this context, there are two strengths regarding a broad definition of social and caring professions in European welfare states. First, it can be adapted to the current reality in different European countries. Second, an inclusive definition makes it possible to incorporate informative examples that would fall outside of a narrow definition.

Content of the book in brief

The chapters in this book connect to four themes that are of current concern to social and caring professionals in Europe facing new demands and expectations: knowledge, reflection and identity; control, regulation and management; collaboration, conflict and competition; and assessment, negotiation and decision making. Below we give a brief introduction to the content of these themes as a way to provide a structured entry to the rest of the book.

Knowledge, reflection and identity in the social and caring welfare professions

The contributions in this section connect to the book's first question: How are social and caring welfare professionals' identities influenced by education, work experience and supervision? A clear or stable professional identity is often regarded as desirable partly because it affects confidence and wellbeing of individual professionals, and partly because it is assumed to affect the opportunities of acting effectively in relation to other professions. Chapters in this section examine professional identity in relation to various aspects of education and work. It is obvious that the basis of professional identity is laid during education, but also that identity can continue to develop throughout a professional career. For this to happen, a key condition is analytical reflection, something that is possible to achieve through supervision.

In Chapter Two, Kåre Heggen and Lars Inge Terum discuss what impact education has on professional identity. They argue that since the formation of professional identity is part of a process of socialisation, they have examined the impact of education, identifying mechanisms that may contribute to the development of professional identity. The chapter shows that professional identity is developed through interactions between different actors as teachers, supervisors and peers. But since tensions often exist within different subjects during an education (for example, psychology and law), as well as between different actors, students have to develop a professional identity through interaction with actors who represent slightly different approaches and traditions. This tension poses a challenge for students in the process of forming a professional identity.

Professional identity is also focus of Chapter Three by Linda Bell, Maria Appel Nissen and Jorunn Vindegg. They argue that construction of professional identity requires experience, analytical reflection and time, and it is a lifelong process of learning, acting and reflecting in education and practice. The construction of professional identity is regarded as an interdependent process relating to interaction, knowledge and values, which cannot be separated when exploring identities of welfare professionals. The authors discuss the construction of professional identity during education, in practice and across different contexts.

Chapter Four also touches on professional identity, but in connection with a discussion on professional supervision and professional autonomy. Here Synnöve Karvinen-Niinikoski, Liz Beddoe, Gillian Ruch and Ming-sum Tsui examine the rapidly growing phenomenon of professional supervision, which has become a central element of several modern professions. The expansion of supervision goes hand in hand with professionalisation processes, as well as with the emergence of new managerial regimes like New Public Management. Supervision can therefore be seen as both an instrument of protecting professional autonomy and an instrument of implying politically and economically conditioned forms of governance or a governmental mentality. But the authors see a potential for 'critically reflective supervision' that can help to recognise and manage the fine balance between the supportive and surveillance or managerial organisational dimensions. A conclusion is that supervision can both contribute to the development of professionals themselves and their field of work.

Control, regulation and management

The chapters in this part of the book connect to the second question: How are social and caring welfare professions affected by governance, regulation and control by the state? A common feature of the chapters in this section concerns the state's impact on welfare professions. From a state perspective, social and caring welfare professions are the actors (street-level bureaucrats) that should implement policy in practice. To ensure this, the state uses various forms of technology for control and audit. From a professional perspective, this is often experienced as decreased autonomy, and increased bureaucracy, which reduces professionals' ability to provide tailor-made services in a flexible way.

The first chapter in this section, Chapter Five, by John Chandler, Elisabeth Berg, Marion Ellison and Jim Barry, discusses the contemporary position of social work in the United Kingdom, and in particular the challenges to what is seen as a managerial-technicist version of social work. The chapter begins with focus on the situation from the 1990s to the present day in which this version of social work takes root and flourishes. The discussion then concentrates on three different routes away from a managerial-technicist social work: the first, reconfiguring professional practice in the direction of evaluation in practice, the second 'reclaiming social work' on the Hackney relationship-based model and the third 'reclaiming social work' in a more radical, highly politicised way. Special attention is devoted to a discussion about of how much autonomy the social workers have in different models, but also what kind of autonomy and for what purpose.

Chapter Six, by Anders Hanberger, Lena Lindgren and Lennart Nygren, concentrates on the key features of auditing and accountability. The authors provide a conceptual framework for studying the interplay of audit and democratic governance in today's audit societies, and they use this framework to analyse how two major audit systems play out in a specific, but major, welfare area, namely the elder care sector in Sweden. The chapter also examines the implications of audit and accountability for elder care policy and governance, and discusses desirable as well as perverse consequences for key actors in the field with a special focus on professionals.

In Chapter Seven, Kazimiera Wódz and Krystyna Faliszek examine how regulation from the state may profoundly shape conditions and practices for welfare profession. Relatively new members of the European Union, such as Poland, often lack a tradition of social work as an integral part of the welfare state. Challenges for such countries are both to educate social workers and to create legislative solutions stipulating the responsibilities and professional jurisdiction of occupational groups dealing with social work. In an effort to achieve this in Poland, the state has introduced guidelines for social services, and making social work a mandatory component in municipal social services. The authors argue that strong regulation and control by the government has resulted in the standardisation of social work. This has curtailed professional autonomy in a manner that is unfavourable to social workers as well as the clients.

Collaboration, conflict and competition

The chapters in this section connect to the third question: How are social and caring welfare professions affected by collaboration, conflict and competition with other welfare professions?

The different contributions show that social and caring welfare professions certainly do not exist in a vacuum; they develop and act in relation to a number of other actors and contextual factors. Several chapters, for example, show that the state can be a very important actor in such a process, as can other competing professional groups. This creates tensions, which sometimes instigate further professionalisation, but may also hamper professionals' everyday practice. A popular idea to overcome such tensions is multi-professional collaboration. However, this is easier said than done, not least since different professions often regard the same problem from viewpoints that are difficult to reconcile.

In Chapter Eight, Ilse Julkunen and Elisabeth Willumsen point to a growing need for different welfare professions to collaborate and coordinate their services so as to respond to service users' complex needs. For example, to solve complex cases, doctors, social workers and therapists often need to develop professional knowledge and skills that facilitate interprofessional collaboration. However, multi- or interprofessional services may give rise to demarcation problems and competition between professions. Using data from child welfare services in Finland and Norway, the chapter examines problems connected to the development of multi-professional services that involves interprofessional boundary crossing and knowledge development.

In Chapter Nine, Eline Thornquist and Hildur Kalman claim that any profession progresses both through interaction and in conflict with adjacent professions. Physiotherapy in Norway is a case in point. Its history is characterised by disputes between physicians and physiotherapists over the division of labour and responsibility. Offering an account of the most important milestones in the history of physiotherapy in Norway, this chapter shows how physiotherapists struggled to become part of the country's health services and how they strove to achieve public authorisation and to allocate to the state – not the medical profession – control over the education of physiotherapists. In this struggle against physicians, physiotherapists searched active support from the state, which turned out be an ally, albeit not an easy one to contend with. The chapter also shows how private and public interests played an important role in this process.

Chapter Ten, by Sabina Pawlas-Czyz, Lars Evertsson and Marek Perlinski, concerns the professional development of social work in Poland after 1989. A close connection to the welfare state has been favourable for the development of many welfare professions. But the state does not always act as an ally. It can push professions in a direction they do not want to go. This is what happened with the social work profession in Poland where the profession and state had different opinions about the jurisdiction of social work. The social work profession claimed jurisdiction for social work with children and families with complex needs, while the state chose to give jurisdiction to a new group of professionals – family assistants. The authors argue that this type of jurisdictional dispute should be framed within a political framework, analysing welfare policies as a structuring link between state and professional jurisdiction. The 'fate' of the social work profession in Poland reflects a lack of bargaining capacity vis-à-vis the state to tie social policies concerning social work with children and families to their jurisdiction.

Chapter Eleven, by Joakim Isaksson and Daniel Törnqvist, deals with how a problem, the use of narcotics, may be defined as both a social and a medical problem, and how different definitions of a problem may cause dilemmas for welfare professions involved in treatment. The chapter examines the implication of the fact that these different problem definitions originate from two different academic disciplines (medicine and social science), and that the social perspective on drug abuse is currently challenged by what some describe as the medicalisation of social problems. The authors argue that welfare professionals need to understand and recognise both these perspectives.

Chapter Twelve, by Witold Mandrysz, Marek Perlinski and Lars Evertsson, concerns the challenges of municipal community work. The chapter focuses on the pros and cons of involving professional social workers, employed in municipal social services, as animators of local community-organised projects in urban, socially and economically disadvantaged residential areas. Such projects aim to promote social development by including inhabitants in the process of improving their own situation. The chapter illustrates that local authorities can face great difficulties when using their own staff as the driving force of local community organising. A major difficulty is that many inhabitants have a negative attitude towards welfare institutions and the local authorities, making them unwilling to cooperate. The fact that the social workers animating the projects work for the local authority therefore complicates the situation. The chapter shows that a number of factors can make it difficult to implement spontaneous social action in the form of local community organisation projects.

Assessment, negotiation and decision making

The contributions in this part of the book connect to the fourth question: How do social and caring welfare professionals, in practice, assess and make decisions in their work with clients and patients? A common notion is that professionals' assessment and decision making is quite rational and based on instrumental use of knowledge. This idea is challenged by four chapters that in different ways discern a number of subtle, dynamic, affective and interactive aspects of professional practice. One aspect of welfare professionals' practice that deserves more attention is negotiation.

Chapter Thirteen, by Rasmus Antoft, Kjeld Høgsbro, Maria Appel Nissen and Søren Peter Olesen, discusses some mostly unnoticed, but crucial, aspects of professional practice among welfare professions. In particular, the chapter examines the informal and strategic forms of negotiations occurring within professional practice and how they relate to various forms of complexity. The text illustrates informal and strategic negotiations by using examples from empirical research on different groups of service users (for example, people with dementia, unemployed people, and families with complex problems). A central assertion is that knowledge about such negotiations is vital in terms of understanding how professional practice is actually conducted and how it works. The authors argue that such knowledge can enhance professional creativity, confidence and the capability to act.

In Chapter Fourteen, Lars Evertsson, Björn Blom, Marek Perlinski and Devin Rexvid ask whether complexity in welfare professionals' work can be handled with standardised professional knowledge. In research, complexity in professional work is often discussed in relation to the professional body of knowledge. There is a tendency to relate professional success, problems and shortcomings to flaws and limitations in the professionals' expert knowledge or use of knowledge. To reduce complexity, overcome problematic situations and achieve best practice, welfare states invest considerable resources in raising professional groups' level of knowledge and use of evidence-based knowledge. Non-medical professions such as social workers are expected to adopt and implement the principles that underpin evidence-based medicine. However, based on two empirical studies of social workers within Swedish social services, this chapter argues that problematic situations and complexity in social work are not always the result of a lack of knowledge; neither are they the result of knowledge not being properly applied. The authors argue that such complex and problematic situations cannot be solved by standardised professional knowledge about interventions and results.

Chapter Fifteen, by Devin Rexvid, examines whom social workers and general practitioners regard as clients, and how they gather information about clients. The two professions have very different approaches. For example, in social work, the applicant and client do not need to be the same person, and social workers put clients in a broad social context to examine whether there are other clients, such as a partner or children, who could be affected by the problem. In comparison, general practitioners concentrate on the medical problem, and ascribe the social relationships of clients as less important. The author argues that the 'traditional' theoretical understanding of professional practice as a linear and rational process consisting of diagnosis, inference and treatment reflects general practitioners' practice as a *mono-client* profession, but not social workers' as a *multi-client* profession.

In Chapter Sixteen, Urban Nothdurfter and Søren Peter Olesen discuss activation work as professional practice. The starting point is that in several European countries there is an increasing trend within social and labour market policy to implement employment-oriented policies. In some countries this turn towards employment has opened up a new professional arena for social workers, so-called employment-oriented social work. The chapter address the challenges that this development has brought to the social work profession, especially how knowledge and decision making is negotiated in relation to clients and other professions within the same policy arena. The chapter is based on Danish, Italian and Austrian data including register data, semi-structured interviews, observations and audio recordings.

The final chapter, by Marek Perlinski, Björn Blom and Lars Evertsson, concentrates on current tendencies, movements and challenges for social and caring welfare professions in Europe. The authors take a 'bird's-eye perspective' to spot a number of key issues and trends from the book's various contributions. The discussion focuses on the position that individual welfare states have in relation to welfare professions, since this is one of the more significant tendencies in the book. The chapter also discusses professionals' identity, conflicts between professions and the role of formal knowledge in social and caring welfare professionals' direct practice.

Countries representing European welfare models

The book includes contributions from eight European countries: Austria, Denmark, Finland, Italy, Norway, Poland, Sweden and the UK. Together they represent five different types of European welfare models: Scandinavian, Continental, Anglo-Saxon, Mediterranean and transitional (Steurer and Hametner, 2013).[3] Having contributions describing different types of European welfare model is a strength since different welfare models affect policies, services and professional practices for social and medical care in different ways.

The majority of contributions cover the Scandinavian welfare model.[4] It can be argued that in this model the ties between the state and its social and caring welfare professions are stronger than in other models. In fact welfare professionals in Nordic countries have been almost exclusively employed by either the state or the local administration and because the voluntary sector in Nordic countries is relatively small, professionals have not been tempted to move into private care.

Such close cooperation with the state has given Nordic social and caring professions relatively strong control and influence over welfare policy making, professional training and working conditions, but the proximity to the state has also made them vulnerable. Today this vulnerability is visible in the Scandinavian countries as they embrace the global trend towards NPM (New Public Management) and EBP (Evidence-Based Practice).

The Nordic contributions may serve as illustrations of how social and caring welfare professions may develop in other countries striving toward a welfare model of the Scandinavian type. Several Asian countries, for example, including China and South Korea, currently use Nordic countries as a model when building up or further developing their welfare systems. This includes development of social and caring welfare professions that is financed and governed by the state.

The ambition is that a mix of chapters specific to some countries and chapters that are more general offers the reader both breadth and depth regarding social and caring professions in European welfare states.

Notes

1. In the late 1800s the German statesman (first chancellor) Otto von Bismarck introduced what has come to be regarded as the world's first welfare state, which aimed to increase worker safety by giving workers a higher status in laws and politics. The programme, which covered sickness insurance, accident insurance, old age and disability insurance, he introduced did not, at that time, exist to any significant extent.
2. Roughly speaking, charity social work started in the latter half of the 1800s, and some form of state-organised social work education began to appear during the first half of the 1900s (e.g. in the UK, USA and Sweden).
3. Previous research has discussed three or four models (see Steurer and Hametner, 2013).
4. Iceland is not represented in this book.

References

Abbott, A. (2014) *The system of professions. An essay on the division of expert labor*, Chicago, IL: University of Chicago Press.

Adams, K., Hean, S., Sturgis, P. and Clark, J.M. (2006) 'Investigating the factors influencing professional identity of first-year health and social care students', *Learning in Health and Social Care*, 5(2): 55-68.

Baldwin, P. (1990) *The politics of social solidarity: Class bases of the European welfare state, 1875-1975*, Cambridge: Cambridge University Press.

Beach, D. (2011) 'Some general developments in the restructuring of education and health care professions in Europe', in I.F. Goodson and S. Lindblad (eds) *Professional knowledge and educational restructuring in Europe*, Rotterdam: Sense Publishers, pp 25-39.

Bergmark, Å. and Lundström, T. (2007) 'Unitarian ideals and professional diversity in social work practice – the case of Sweden', *European Journal of Social Work*, 10(1): 55-72.

Bijak, J., Kicinger, A. and Kupiszewski, M. (2013) 'International migration scenarios for 27 European countries, 2002–2052', in M. Kupiszewski (ed) *International migration and the future of populations and labour in Europe*, Dordrecht: Springer, pp 75-92.

Blom, B. (2004) 'Specialization in social work practice', *Journal of Social Work*, 4(1): 25-46.

Conrad, P. and Potter, D. (2000) 'From hyperactive children to ADHD adults: observations on the expansion of medical categories', *Social Problems*, 47(4): 559-82.

Conrad, P. and Schneider, J.W. (2010) *Deviance and medicalization: From badness to sickness*, Philadelphia, PA: Temple University Press.

Ek, A.C., Ideland, M., Jönsson, S. and Malmberg, C. (2013) 'The tension between marketisation and academisation in higher education', *Studies in Higher Education*, 38(9): 1305-18.

Ellett, A.J., Ellis, J.I., Westbrook, T.M. and Dews, D. (2007) 'A qualitative study of 369 child welfare professionals' perspectives about factors contributing to employee retention and turnover', *Children and Youth Services Review*, 29(2): 264-81.

Freidson, E. (1970) *Professional dominance: The social structure of medical care*, New York, NY: Atherton Press.

Freidson, E. (2001) *Professionalism: The third logic*, Cambridge: Polity Press.

Forsell, A. and Ivarsson Westerberg, A. (2014) *Administrationssamhället* [The administration society], Lund: Studentlitteratur.

Greenwood, E. (1957) 'Attributes of a profession', *Social Work*, 2(3): 45-55.

Guzman, R.U. (2012) *Managed care: An investigation of the relationship between the dimensions of de-professionalization and physician satisfaction*, Minneapolis, MN: Capella University.

Healy, K. (2009) 'A case of mistaken identity. The social welfare professions and New Public Management', *Journal of Sociology*, 45(4): 401-18.

Jessen, J.T. (2011) *Forvaltning av velferd: Yrkesutøvelse i møte med byråkrati og brukere* [Administration of welfare: Professional work in the encounter with bureaucracy and clients], Trondheim: NTNU.

Johnson, T. (1972) *Professions and power*, London: Macmillan.

Kim, E.H., Linker, D.T., Coumar, A., Dean, L.S., Matsen F.A and Kim Y. (2011) 'Factors affecting acceptance of a web-based self-referral system', *IEEE Transactions on Information Technology in Biomedicine*, 15(2): 344-47.

Korpi, W. and Palme, J. (1998) 'The paradox of redistribution and strategies of equality: welfare state institutions, inequality, and poverty in the Western countries', *American Sociological Review*, 63(5): 661-87.

Kuhnle, S. (ed) (2000) *Survival of the European welfare state*, London: Routledge.

Laffin, M. and Entwistle, T. (2000) 'New problems, old professions? The changing national world of the local government professions', *Policy & Politics*, 28(2): 207-20.

Manthorpe, J., Moriarty, J., Hussein, S., Stevens, M. and Sharpe, E. (2015) 'Content and purpose of supervision in social work practice in England: views of newly qualified social workers, managers and directors', *British Journal of Social Work*, 45(1): 52-68.

Mieg, H. A. (2008) 'Professionalisation and professional identities of environmental experts: the case of Switzerland', *Environmental Sciences*, 5(1): 41-51.

Molander, A. and Terum, L.I. (2008) 'Profesjonsstudier: en introduksjon' [Studies of professions: an introduction], in A. Molander and L.I. Terum (eds) *Profesjonsstudier* [Studies of professions], Oslo: Universitetsforlaget, pp 13-27.

Power, M. (1999) *The audit society: Rituals of verification*, Oxford: Oxford University Press.

Quadagno, J. (1987) 'Theories of the welfare state', *Annual Review of Sociology*, 13: 109-28.

Rexvid, D., Blom, B., Evertsson, L. and Forssén, A. (2012) 'Risk reduction technologies in general practice and social work', *Professions and Professionalism*, 2(2).

Rose, J. (2011) 'Dilemmas of inter-professional collaboration: can they be resolved?', *Children & Society*, 25(2): 151-63.

Safatti-Larson, M. (1977) *The rise of professionalism*, Berkeley, CA: Berkeley University Press.

Segev, N., Boehm, A. and Vigoda-Gadot, E. (2012) 'Organizational and personal antecedents in adaptation of market-orientation in the public sector. An empirical study of local municipal social-welfare agencies', in L. Matei and J.L. Vazquez-Burguete (eds) *Permanent Study Group: Public and Nonprofit Marketing, Proceedings*, Bucharest: Editura Economica, pp 61-78.

Steurer, R. and Hametner, M. (2013) 'Objectives and indicators in sustainable development strategies: similarities and variances across Europe', *Sustainable Development*, 21(4): 224-41.

Part 1
Knowledge, reflection and identity in the social and caring welfare professions

TWO

The impact of education on professional identity

Kåre Heggen and Lars Inge Terum

Introduction

The role of a professional social worker requires knowledge, skills, practical wisdom and certain norms and standards. Professional practice depends on the ability to combine these elements. Professional identity refers to social workers' motivation for doing good work and their identification with the profession. The formation of professional identity is closely connected to socialisation and is a part of a dynamic process of professional development. The aim of this chapter is to examine the impact of social work education on professional identity.

In the literature on professional education, the concept 'professional identity' is frequently used, but in a variety of different meanings and contexts (Beijaard et al, 2004; Sims, 2011; Johnson et al, 2012; Wiles, 2012; Trede et al, 2013) and remains 'fuzzy' and 'elusive' and with 'no explicit definition' (Lamote and Engels, 2010, p 4; Sims, 2011, p 266). Professional identity refers to '... the principles, intentions, characteristics and experiences by which an individual defines him or herself in a professional role' (McSweeney, 2012, p 367), as a lens through which to evaluate, learn and make sense of practice (Trede et al, 2013) or the '... perception of her/himself in the context of nursing practice' (Steinbock-Hult, 1985). In some authors' work, the perception is that identity as a professional primarily is developed in the community of practice to which one belongs and where knowledge from outside has a minor influence on professional identity (Wenger, 1998). In this approach, a strong professional identity will be shaped and reinforced by strong and stable communities and social processes generated within them (Henkel, in Reid et al, 2008).

Since the formation of professional identity is part of a process of socialisation, we intend to examine the impact of education, identifying mechanisms that may contribute to the development of professional identity. What can be learned from a literature review and what do we suggest might be important mechanisms? The focus is on social work education, but owing to a more extensive research literature, nursing and teacher education will also, to some extent, be included.

First, we introduce the literature on the formation of professional identity and the impact of professional education. Second, we develop the argument that the organisation of education and the interactions between students and teachers/supervisors are of crucial importance for the development of professional identity.

Research methods

In order to find relevant and important literature, we searched for articles and book chapters in Bibsys advanced search, Academic Search Elite, Article First and Eric. Key terms were 'professional identity', 'professional education', 'social work identity' and 'social work education'. This search gave us more than 260 journal articles and book chapters, and we read the abstracts. About 60 papers were assessed to be relevant to our investigation and therefore read more systematically. Most of the selected papers investigate and analyse social work and professional identity, although some of them discuss teacher or nursing education. A few of them analyse the impact of higher education on professional identity in general. Finally, about 25 articles/book chapters were selected and analysed for this study, among them articles from 20 international journals.

Formation of professional identity

According to social identity theory, people tend to classify themselves into various categories and identities that refer to a person's belonging to certain human values. As such, social identification provides a partial answer to the question 'Who am I?', and the answer is given in relation to a category (Ashforth and Mael, 1989). In addition, scholars have argued that identification with a profession refers to an ongoing process that is dynamic and relational. It is not only the answer to the question of 'Who am I?' but also the answer to the question of 'Who do I want to become?' (Beijaard et al, 2004, pp 122-3). It refers less to something that professionals have and more to a process that involves making sense of oneself as a professional. Understood this way, formation of professional identity is closely connected to professional socialisation.

In a structural-functional perspective, professional socialisation has been interpreted as internalisation of values and the development of an identity as a member of a profession. Professional socialisation is pictured as an orderly and smooth process during which students' internalise roles, norms and values (Vågan, 2009). Fostering professional identity is, however, probably more complicated than adopting certain traits, values and competences (Wiles, 2012, p 864). It is alternatively described as a non-linear process (Barretti, 2004; Krejsler, 2005), rather than a role achieved through passive acceptance.

An alternative approach, based on the perspective of symbolic interactionism, looks at professional socialisation as the creation of a professional role – a process characterised by conflicts and contradictions, rather than of harmony and uniqueness. Professional socialisation is understood as a recurring process of adjustment to various expectations and demands. A crucial issue is how such potential tensions influence the creation of the identification with social work as an occupation and a profession. This approach has also been termed the reaction approach because students are interpreted as active and conscious agents whose professional identity is being developed in their interactions with teachers and fellow students (Barretti, 2004).

In a structural-functional perspective, professional identity is understood as a collective concept, referring to a common identity for the profession, while the reaction approach focuses on the individual process, emphasising that each individual has to create and develop their role as social worker (Jenkins, 2004; Wiles, 2012, p 864). In a way, they are competing perspectives; however, they also have some aspects of professional identity in common.

Professional identity refers to a particular profession, which means that identity as a social worker is different from identity as a teacher, although both represent professional identity. At the same time, the development of professional identity refers to a process on an individual level: '... who one is as a person is so much interwoven with who one acts as professional, both sides cannot be separated' (Lamote and Engels, 2010, p 4). We refer to Sachs' description in Beauchamp and Thomas (2009, p 178) where professional identity is explained as a developing framework about how 'to be', how 'to act' and how to 'understand' as a professional. The development of professional identity is understood as a dynamic, ongoing process where personal history, social interactions and psychological and cultural factors have an influence. Professional identity includes who a person is, but also what kind of a professional they want to become.

Impact of education

In the literature review, we analytically differentiate between assumptions based on professional education and identity formation expressed in general theories and empirical evidence of the role of education in the development of professional identity.

Assumptions

In research on professions, education has generally been ascribed an important role in the shaping of students' identification with future occupations (Merton, 1957; Parsons, 1978; Freidson, 2001; Barretti, 2004). According to Freidson (2001), professional education '... contributes to the development of commitment to the occupation as a life career and to a shared identity, a feeling of community or solidarity among those who have passed through it' (Freidson, 2001, p 84).

Professional education involves dealing not only with knowledge and skills, but also with attitudes, values and aspirations (Pascarella and Terenzini, 2005, p 6). In his conceptualisation of professionalism, Sullivan (2005) ascribes education an important role in the development of professional identity. A common challenge of professional education is how to handle the complex composition of analytic thinking, skilful practice and wise judgment and to integrate these aspects of expertise into a consistent professional identity (Sullivan et al, 2007). These aspects are described as the three apprenticeships – the intellectual or cognitive, the apprenticeship of skilful practice, and that of wise professional judgment. Sullivan argues that the lack of integration of these elements is the greatest challenge of professional education (2005, p 196). Students with little or no direct exposure to practical experiences are one of the challenges. Another challenge could be academic educational models' 'abstraction from actual application of knowledge to practice' (p 197). An impact of this could be too large a distance to students' moral and practical formation. The pedagogical challenge for education is to promote the integration of analytical and practical competencies required of professional practice. It is the integrity or the synthesis of the three apprenticeships that develops professionalism. However, Sullivan describes the third as the one 'through which the students' professional self can be most broadly explored and developed' (p 209), and continues: '... the third apprenticeship of professional identity has to precede and interpenetrate the learning of formal analytic knowledge in the first apprenticeship and the development of skilled practice in the second' (pp 253–4).

Most professional education involves the organisation and teaching of a vast number of subjects by teachers and supervisors who represent different perspectives, traditions and approaches. Professional education is infrequently uniform and paradigmatic. Tensions exist within and between subjects as well as between faculty members and supervisors during placements. In this situation, students have to develop a professional identity as social workers through interaction with peers, faculty members and supervisors who represent slightly different approaches and traditions.

Empirical evidence

Even though social work education is expected to be important in professional socialisation, empirical research on this subject is limited (Barretti, 2004; Lishman, 2012). Nevertheless some studies have examined the impact of social work education on students' attitudes, values, preferences and so on (Pike, 1994; Barretti, 2004; Weiss et al, 2004; Limb and Organista, 2006; Kaufman et al, 2012). The general picture is mixed – some indicate a significant impact, but others do not. The main reasons for such a divergence could include the variation in research designs, with small samples and studies often limited to a single school of social work (Pike, 1994; Barretti, 2004), or the lack of longitudinal data and design (Weiss et al, 2004). Johnson and colleagues emphasise that the qualifying process and the transition to practice means that the students undergo a constant reshaping of professional identity. This illustrates the need for longitudinal studies to investigate empirical effects (Johnson et al, 2012).

Trede and colleagues (2013) conducted a review of relevant higher education literature on the development of professional identities. Preparation at university includes learning about professional roles, understanding workplace cultures, commencing the professional socialization process and educating oneself towards citizenship – all which contribute to the development of professional identities. It may be the integration of professional, personal and social identities that '... is manifested when students see the relevance of what they are doing and learning, and when they feel valued for what they know and do' (p 376). One conclusion from the review is that a combination of education and students' work experiences shape the development of a professional identity, although universities seem to play a relatively weak role in this regard once students engage in learning in the workplace. An implication for universities seems to be that 'the effective use of experiences that lead to heightened self-awareness and deeper understanding of practice appear to be key concerns in professional identity development' (p 378).

Lamote and Engels (2010) conducted a cross-sectional investigation on students' emerging professional identities. They find that the development of professional identity fluctuates throughout the education process – and is vulnerable in the face of practice. Their advice, which reflects that of Trede and colleagues, is to invite new students to explore and articulate their perceptions, to create opportunities to experience the complexity of practice and provide systematic support to these learning processes (p 16). They also refer to the effect of the knowledge base, which is seen as relevant for practice by both individuals and the profession as a whole.

Adams and colleagues (2006) investigated factors influencing professional identity of first-year health and social care students. One of their findings is that a degree of professional identity is already evident before students begin their professional education, even if the extent varied across the professions. Significant predictors were gender, profession, and previous work experience in health and social care environments, as well as knowledge of the problems and understanding of teamworking (p 55). Beauchamp and Thomas, studying teacher training, also focus on the meaning of the educational programme. Even if important development of professional identity takes place later on, the educational programme plays a key role in highlighting the need for students to develop an identity and the ongoing shifts that will occur in that identity (Beauchamp and Thomas, 2009, p 186).

In a qualitative study of Master's students in social work, Osteen (2011) underlines the development and integration of professional values as a main dimension in professional identity. He makes a distinction between personal values, important motivators for students' decision to start social work education, and the acquisition of core values unique to the profession. During the students' education, value conflicts between personal and professional values were found to be a common occurrence. Osteen concludes that for many students 'the educational process reaffirmed their personal values and strengthened their commitment to professional social work values. For some students the educational process challenged them and resulted in the desire to incorporate professional values more fully in their personal life. A third way the program impacted value systems was to reveal value incongruity' (Osteen, 2011, p 433).

McSweeney (2012) conducted a qualitative study of part-time social care students throughout their three-year Bachelor's education. She found factors that encourage students' identity, especially 'pedagogical strategies that make use of students' experiences, but also locate these in a theoretical context …'. This involves more than a narrow focus on the workplace (p 377). The author emphasises how important it is to integrate student and work identity and not to keep them separate.

Elsewhere, Shlomo and colleagues (2012) analysed the development of professional identity among 176 third-year student social workers at an Israeli university. The influence of three sets of resources were investigated – organisational, personal and environmental. The impact of education was in their analysis especially connected to how satisfied students were with supervision throughout their education. Their conclusion was that satisfaction with supervision contributes strongly to the development of a professional identity. They also suggest further examination of the relationship between student and supervisor. A weakness with this study, however, is the cross-sectional character of the examination. A longitudinal design would probably have given it greater validity.

Beddoe (2011) analyses social workers in healthcare and the links between knowledge, credentials and a sense of professional identity. Her investigation was conducted in New Zealand, where social work has been 'a "guest" under the benign control of the medical and nursing profession' (p 29), and where the development of professional identity is, for that reason, very complex. Nevertheless, Beddoe found that professional identity develops over time and involves attitudes, values, knowledge, beliefs and skills shared with others within the profession. She also found that social workers sought to enhance their professional capital and identity through education and the achievement of higher credentials.

Earls Larrison and Korr (2013) use Shulman's concept of signature pedagogies, which in their eyes involves the interpretation of practitioner knowledge, performative action and awareness, which emphasises the development of the professional self (p 194). What is important in their approach is that social work's signature pedagogies involve central forms of teaching and learning in classrooms, and 'through the relational teaching-learning encounters and interactions between and among social work students and educators' (p 197). An earlier investigation by Larrison (cited in Larrison and Korr, 2013) reveals that the relational investment between social work educators and their students influenced the students' understanding of how one's use of self was implemented in practice – relations that helped to integrate their personal and professional identities (p 202).

Terum and Heggen (2015) used a longitudinal approach (StudData)[1] to measure the impact of the education on professional identity. The concept 'professional identity' is empirically measured using a range of indicators relating to students' identification with the profession, their choice of education and the occupation of social worker. The students answered the same set of questions at the start and at the end of their three-year education, and two professions – social work and nursing – are compared. Three independent variables were developed: teacher–student interaction, supervisor–student interaction and peer interaction.

The analysis indicates that professional identification is established at an early stage of education; that the level of professional identification at entrance largely predicts the level at the end of education; and that education has a positive impact on students' professional identification.

Because students are interpreted as active agents in the formation of professional identification (Terum and Heggen, 2015), 'interactions' are emphasised. In this study, teacher–student interaction and interaction with supervisors at placement affects professional identification. In accordance with previous research, this indicates that students who experience support and feedback from teachers and who have confidence in the supervisors' competence express a stronger dedication to and identification with the profession. However, not all students perceive supervisors as good role models or have teachers with the ability to provide good and relevant feedback. This is not only an effect of how teachers and supervisors act and perform but also an effect of how students act and react. This indicates that students interpret and experience teachers and supervisors differently.

Our conclusion so far is that research on the role of social work education is inconsistent, although there are some indications that workplace, and, to some degree, higher education, are important factors in students' development of professional identity.

Coherence

In view of the non-paradigmatic character of social work education, the concept of 'coherence' is interesting. This refers to the degree of internal connection or, alternatively, fragmentation in the programme – the way that different parts of education are related to each other and to future professional work (Grossman et al, 2008). In this analysis, we include our own work, which focuses on the interactions between student and teacher, theory and practice, and student and supervisor, along with that of our peers (Heggen and Terum, 2013), and some international studies that analyse the relationship between coherence in educational programmes and students' professional identity.

Even if the concept of coherence is quite new, and was developed as an analytic concept only in recent decades, much of the content is quite old. The so-called theory–practice debate is important, as it has featured in discussions about professional education for more than a hundred years, even if it has intensified in recent years.

One understanding of coherent education is a more harmonised education. This is not our understanding. Coherence in our view also means education characterised by sensible tensions and negotiations. In the following definition in support of the harmonisation perspective, here connected to teacher training, coherence is understood as '… shared understanding among faculty and in the manner in which opportunities to learn have been arranged (organisationally, logistically) to achieve a common goal – that of educating professional teachers with the knowledge, skills, and dispositions necessary to more effectively teach diverse students …' (Tatto, 1996, p 176).

We have two objections to this definition of coherence. The first is that shared understanding among faculty members (teachers, practice supervisors and other educational staff) is described as a possible and even desirable purpose in professional education. A more realistic approach is probably that different members of the faculty in different subjects or disciplines will represent different and often contrasting views. In a coherent education, such different views and perspectives have to be managed in constructive ways, rather than being eliminated (Stjernø, 1996, p 42). Our second objection is that Tatto's definition is concerned about common understandings between faculty members, while the important question is how students understand and develop their understanding and motivation. In our approach, what is most important is how students manage to see their qualification process as coherent and meaningful. Coherent qualification is perceived as learning processes where students take part in discussions and negotiations and on that basis develop their knowledge, practical skills and professional identity.

We find that Grimen (2008) grasps these important dimensions of coherence. Grimen claims that for a professional education to be meaningful and coherent, it should create practical synthesis out of teaching and training. While you can develop meaningful coherence in disciplines like physics and chemistry through theoretical synthesis, this is not possible in a professional education, where the curriculum consists of subjects and disciplines without a logical internal connection. Here academic content can make a synthesis only when the parts are directed towards, and integrated, in practical tasks that are to be performed in this profession – practical synthesis. The core of Grimen's understanding, as we see it, is that students in a professional education need experiences with guided practice to apply theoretical knowledge from relevant theories. This could be seen as a precondition for students developing a 'feel' for how to exert professional performance, what we may call professional identity.

Coherence and professional identity

In our systematic review of academic publications about professional identity, especially about social workers, we have found very few that investigate the impact of coherence and how well the different parts of training and qualifying for professional work is integrated – on development of professional identity. The lack of longitudinal investigations of this question – which is probably the preferred methodological approach for identifying the relationship between education and professional identity – is striking. One example of a longitudinal approach, however, is McSweeney's study (2012, described earlier), which followed 15 social work students through their three-year education, and underlines the importance of integrating students' work experiences and their introduction to the theoretical context, to foster their professional identity.

One investigation uses the concept 'coherence' (Shlomo et al, 2012). These authors' concept is, however, 'sense of coherence', as a personal resource connected to Antonovsky's conceptualisation. The three important dimensions in Antonovsky's concept are comprehensibility, manageability and meaningfulness (Antonovsky, 1987). Used as an individual concept, the authors found that it had no impact on students' development of professional identity. A possible problem with this conceptualisation related to our research question is that sense of coherence in this project is not directed against the educational programme, but is related to 'a global orientation students have about their lives and what they can expect to happen' (Shlomo et al, 2012, p 243).

Through a cross-sectional investigation of 176 third-year social work students, Shlomo and colleagues (2012) investigated the eventual influence of three types of resource on professional identity: organisational, personal and environmental. The personal resources were 'emphatic behaviour', 'self-differentiation' and 'sense of coherence'. The organisational resource was 'satisfaction with supervision', while the environmental resources was students' value orientation. Their conclusion was that satisfaction with supervision had a great impact on students' professional identity, while 'sense of coherence' had no significant impact (p 249).

In the context of this chapter – the impact of education on students' professional identity – we have two objections to the investigation of Shlomo and colleagues. The first is the cross-sectional methodology, data collected with the use of a questionnaire distributed among third-year students. We find this to be problematic in attempting to measure the effects of educational processes due to the lack of a longitudinal approach. The second objection is the content of 'sense of coherence'. In our view it is difficult to investigate the impact of education when this is defined as a 'global' concept and not directed to the educational context and whether the students experienced a coherent education or not.

In a study of professional education by Heggen and Terum (2013), students' sense of coherence in education was found to have a significant impact on dedication to and identification with the professions. The study analysed longitudinal survey data collected from students in colleges for teaching, nursing and social work. The data were collected in the first and third years of education. The main conclusion is that the content and organisation of education matter, indicating that it is possible to plan and organise educational programmes in ways that strengthen students' motivation and identity with their future work.

Three of four investigated aspects of coherence have significant impact on identity and dedication, even after controlling for identification at entry to the education; theory–practice interaction, peer interaction and supervisor interaction (not teacher–student interaction). The main finding is that professional education contributes when students experience a clear relationship between schoolwork and fieldwork as well as satisfactory interactions with peers and supervisors. This conclusion should encourage teachers to strengthen such factors in education programmes.

Conclusion

The aim of professional education is to achieve both cognitive and affective aims that deal with values, motivation and attitudes. In this chapter, the intention has been to discuss the impact of professional education on the formation of identity. Our first conclusion is that the impact of professional education on students' dedication to and identification with the profession needs to be examined more thoroughly. This requires more longitudinal data and sophisticated analysis.

Second, professional identity is developed through interactions between students, teachers, supervisors and peers. Due to the non-paradigmatic character of social work education, internal coherence is an important factor. In addition, because training involves both classroom and workplace learning, it is important to acknowledge that tensions might exist within subjects as well as between faculty members and supervisors at placement. In this situation, students have to develop a professional identity as social workers through interaction with peers, faculty members and supervisors who represent slightly different approaches and traditions. The main challenge is not the non-paradigmatic character of social work, but rather how this fragmentation is dealt with and experienced by students. The knowledge about these processes, and how they affect the formation of professional identity, is incomplete.

Note

1 StudData is a longitudinal survey, developed at the Centre for the Study of Professions, Oslo and Akershus University College. StudData includes four student cohorts in approximately 20 professional programmes (for nurses, social workers, teachers and physicians) and data are collected from each respondent four times; at the beginning and end of education, and three and six years after graduation; see www.hioa.no/eng/Forskning-og-utvikling/Hva-forsker-HiOA-paa/FoU-SPS/prosjekter/StudData.

References

Adams, K., Hean, S., Sturgis, P. and Clark, J.M. (2006) 'Investigating the factors influencing professional identity of first-year health and social care students', *Learning in Health and Social Care*, 5(2): 55-68.

Antonovsky, A. (1987) *Unravelling the mystery of health*, San Fransisco, CA: Jossey-Bass.

Ashforth, B.E. and Mael, F. (1989) 'Social identity theory and the organization', *Academy of Management Review*, 14(1): 20-39.

Barretti, M. (2004) 'What do we know about the professional socialization of our students?', *Journal of Social Work Education*, 40(2): 255-83.

Beddoe, L. (2011) 'Health and social work: professional identity and knowledge', *Qualitative Social Work*, 12(1): 24-40.

Beijaard, D., Meijer, P. and Verloop, N. (2004) 'Reconsidering research on teachers' professional identity', *Teaching and Teacher Education*, 20(2): 107-28.

Beauchamp, C. and Thomas, L. (2009) 'Understanding teacher identity: an overview of issues in the literature and implications for teacher education', *Cambridge Journal of Education*, 39(2): 175-89.

Earls Larrison, T. and Korr, W.S. (2013) 'Does social work have a signature pedagogy?', *Journal of Social Work Education*, 49(2): 194-206.

Freidson, E. (2001) *Professionalism. The third logic*, Oxford: Polity.

Grimen, H. (2008) 'Profesjon og kunnskap' [Profession and knowledge], in A. Molander and L.I. Terum (eds) *Profesjonsstudier* [*Studies of professions*], Oslo: Universitetsforlaget, pp 71-86.

Grossman, P., Hammerness, K., McDonald, M. and Ronfeldt, M. (2008) 'Constructing Coherence', *Journal of Teacher Education*, 59(4): 273-87.

Heggen, K. and Terum, L.I. (2013) 'Coherence in professional education: does it foster dedication and identification?', *Teaching in Higher Education*, 18(6): 656-69.

Jenkins, R. (2004) *Social identity*, London: Routledge.

Johnson, M., Cowin, L.S., Wilson, I. and Young, H. (2012) 'Professional identity and nursing: contemporary theoretical developments and future research challenges', *International Nursing Review*, 59(4): 562-69.

Kaufman, R., Segal-Engelchin, D. and Huss, E. (2012) 'Transitions in first-year students' initial practice orientation', *Journal of Social Work Education*, 48(2): 337-59.

Krejsler, J. (2005) 'Professions and their identities: how to explore professional development among (semi-) professions', *Scandinavian Journal of Educational Research*, 29(4): 335-57.

Lamote, C. and Engels, N. (2010) 'The development of student teachers' professional identity', *European Journal of Teacher Education*, 33(1): 3-18.

Limb, G.E. and Organista, K.C. (2006) 'Change between entry and graduation in MSW student views on social work's traditional mission, career motivation, and practice preferences: Caucasian, student of color, and American Indian group comparisons', *Journal of Social Work Education*, 42(2): 269-89.

Lishman, J. (2012) *Social work education and training, Research Highlights 54*, London: Jessica Kingsley.

McSweeney, F. (2012) 'Student, practitioner, or both? Separation and integration of identities in professional social care education', *Social Work Education*, 31(3): 364-82.

Merton, R.K. (1957) *Social theory and social structure*, New York, NY: Free Press.

Osteen, P.J. (2011) 'Motivations, values, and conflict resolution: students' integration of personal and professional identities', *Journal of Social Work Education*, 47(3): 423-44.

Parsons, T. (1978) *Action theory and the human condition*, New York, NY: Free Press.

Pascarella, E.T. and Terenzini, P.T. (2005) *How college affects students. A third decade of research* (vol 2), San Francisco, CA: Jossey-Bass.

Pike, C.K. (1994) 'Development of the social work values inventory', University of Alabama, Dissertation Abstracts International, 55(1), 1696A.

Reid, A., Dahlgren, L.O., Petocz, P. and Dahlgren, M.A. (2008) 'Identity and engagement for professional formation', *Studies in Higher Education*, 33(6): 729-42.

Shlomo, S.B., Levy, D. and Itzhaky, H. (2012) 'Development of professional identity among social work students: contributing factors', *The Clinical Supervisor*, 31(2), 240-55.

Sims, D. (2011) 'Reconstructing professional identity for professional and interprofessional practice: a mixed methods study of joint training programmes in learning disability nursing and social work', *Journal of Interprofessional Care*, 25(4): 265-71.

Steinbock-Hult, B. (1985) 'Yrkesidentitet' [Work identity], *Sairaanhoitaja*, 2, 9-14.

Stjernø, S. (1996) ´Har profesjonsutdanningene felleskomponenter?' [Do professional education have common elements?], in V. Bunkholdt, A.G. Eritsland and K. Jensen (eds) *Kunnskap og omsorg. Sosialisering og skikkethet I profesjonsutdanningene* [*Knowledge and care. Socialization and aptitude in professional education*], Oslo: Tano.

Sullivan, W.M. (2005) *Work and integrity. The crisis and promise of professionalism in America*, San Francisco, CA: Jossey-Bass.

Sullivan, W.M., Colby, A., Wegner, J.W., Bond, L. and Shulman, L.S. (2007) *Educating lawyers: Preparation for the profession of law*, San Francisco, CA: Jossey-Bass.

Tatto, M.T. (1996) 'Examining values and beliefs about teaching diverse students: understanding the challenges for teacher education', *Educational Evaluation and Policy Analysis*, 18(2): 155-80.

Terum, L.I. and Heggen, K. (2015) 'Identification with the social work profession: the impact of education', *British Journal of Social Work*, doi:1093/bjsw/bcv026.

Trede, F., Macklin, R and Bridges, D. (2013) 'Professional identity development: a review of the higher education literature', *Studies in Higher Education*, 37(3): 365-84.

Vågan, A. (2009) *Physicians in the making*, Oslo: Oslo University College.

Weiss, I., Gal, J. and Cnaan, R.A. (2004) 'Social work education as professional socialization', *Journal of Social Service Research*, 31(1): 13-31.

Wenger, A. (1998) *Communities of practice. Learning, meaning, and identity*, Cambridge: Cambridge University Press.

Wiles, F. (2012) 'Not easily put into a box: constructing professional identity', *Social Work Education: The International Journal*, 32(7): 854-66.

THREE

The construction of professional identity in social work: experience, analytical reflection and time

Linda Bell, Maria Appel Nissen and Jorunn Vindegg

Introduction

In their journeys towards becoming and developing as professionals, social work students and practitioners form a range of beliefs and attitudes about the profession. Norms and values are embedded in various knowledge bases, crucial for work performance, and are also noticeable in social and educational policies framing professional practice. Several components influence the professional development of every practitioner. Simultaneously, professionals develop understanding of their professional boundaries and how they may interact with others through interprofessional cooperation. Their set of beliefs, attitudes and understanding about their roles, within the work context, is generally referred to as their 'professional identity'. We consider professional identity and its construction as 'a lifelong process', influencing the kinds of knowledge demanded in education and in practice. This process of construction itself implies that professional identity is an 'interactional accomplishment' that can 'only be understood as process, as "being" or "becoming", never a final or settled matter' (Jenkins, 2004, p 6).

From this point of departure, it is crucial to investigate how these constructing processes proceed in different fields and at different levels. This chapter aims to provide a contribution to filling gaps in understanding these reflective processes by demonstrating how various components are involved in the process of identity construction. Drawing on several examples from Denmark, England and Norway, we identify how this process involves the construction of *experience*, *analytical reflection* and *time* across the field of *education* and *practice* and in reflection over *theory and practice*. This process of constructing professional identity is characterised by sensitivity towards interactional and contextual complexity including openness to the ambiguity of knowledge. This contrasts with approaches that presume professional identity and practice are constructed unambiguously. Therefore a major point of the chapter is that social and educational policies offering a simplistic approach can be problematic, by ignoring the complex construction of professional identity. We will discuss this issue at the end of the chapter with reference to the current focus on evidence-based knowledge and practice.

The construction of professional identity

Jenkins (2004) points out in his theoretical discussion of approaches to social identity derived from social psychology (for example Robinson, 1996) and sociology/anthropology (for example Barth, 2000) that individuals and collectivities produce and reproduce 'identity' through discourse, narrative and representation, as well as through practical and material processes of identification. For example, we argue here that social workers use their practical experience as well as analytical reflection to construct a sense of identity as an individual professional as well as a professional group or collective. Both experience and reflection are underpinned by time in significant ways as we will see later. Jenkins also points to the significance of 'external' identification by others in the construction of such identity/ies.

Currently there are many debates relating professionalism fairly straightforwardly to evidence-based practice and research (Webb, 2001; Gilgun, 2005). By focusing on construction of professional identity in social work, identifying in detail the knowledge, values and interactions that can occur within professional practice, and during professional education/socialisation, we aim to present a more sophisticated understanding of how welfare professionals, and in particular, social workers, develop their identity/ies in different contexts. There is even a possibility that social workers may be constructing several different kinds of professional identity related to different specialities. How identity/ies emerge during interactions in professional practice and education for practice is related not only to 'evidence-based' sources but also to wider sources of knowledge, as well as to concerns for professional values and ethics (Bell, 2015).

These processes begin during professional education where, with support from educators, students begin to construct a professional identity. Trede and colleagues' review (2012) concludes by demonstrating the dynamic transformative nature of professional identity development, personal sense making and student participation. Collaborative, dialogic learning from practice enables and facilitates professional identity development. Furthermore, the authors found a strong emphasis on the individual learner, although collective learning was also discussed. Tensions between personal and professional values and structural and power influences were identified for further debate and investigation. Moreover, the authors emphasised the need for further exploration into the meaning of professional identity development.

Trede and colleagues limited their review to higher education research, but call attention to the vast body of relevant literature not specifically linked to higher education. As an example, Herbert and Stuart Dreyfus (1986) developed a model of skills acquisition. They describe a five-stage process during which the individual's practical competence is developed. Stages one to three describe development from novice to competent, the last two stages the proficient and the expert. Progression is thus from rigid adherence to rules to an intuitive mode of reasoning based on tacit knowledge. A criticism of this model has been provided by Gobet and Chassy (2009), who also propose an alternative theory of intuition, suggesting there is no empirical evidence for stages in the development of expertise. Also, while the model argues that analytic thinking does not play any role with experts, who act only intuitively, there is evidence elsewhere that experts often carry out relatively slow problem solving. We fully agree with these objections and would emphasise the analytical position of professionals. Previous work shows what is involved in construction of everyday career identities, for example, of professionals involved in work-based training activities (Bell, 2007).

Donald Schön (1983) challenged practitioners to reconsider the role of technical knowledge versus 'artistry' in developing professional excellence. Through a feedback loop of experience, learning and practice, professionals can continually improve their work, whether educational or not, and become a 'reflective practitioner'. Chris Argyris and Donald Schön (1996) also maintained that organizations and individuals should be flexible and incorporate lessons learned throughout life, known as organizational learning. However, as Schön points out, processes of reflection required for learning are not initiated automatically. A crucial question is what enables professional learning and identity building.

It is generally acknowledged that professional identity is closely related to use of knowledge. Some even view professional identity as synonymous with knowledge, arguing professional knowledge is genuinely constituted *differentially* – not only on the basis of knowledge based on action and experience but also incorporating more abstract forms of knowledge including theory – and as reflection on and recombination of these different forms into a professional knowledge base suitable for solving problems in practice (Oettingen, 2007; Nissen, 2010). If so, reflection can be viewed as an analytical endeavour, also representing an attempt to reconcile the often contested relationship between theory and practice. We argue that complexity of problems and forms of knowledge at play in contemporary professional practice require professionals to uphold both a sense of 'lived experience' as well as knowledge of how actions and experiences can be understood and explained in a more abstract and thus general sense. In practice it takes time to develop such analytical competence – indeed it is a lifelong process. To illustrate this and explore the 'components' of the process of developing professional identity, experience, time and analytical reflection, we draw on examples from recent studies.

Experience: ambiguity and narrative constructions

A Norwegian study illuminates what kind of knowledge professional social workers exploit as well as construct in their daily practices (Vindegg, 2011). Forty-one qualitative interviews were carried out with social workers, parents and children cooperating in child welfare departments in various municipalities. An analytical gaze was directed towards how social workers talked about parents who have children referred to and in need of help from the child welfare system, that is, how social categories as 'mother' and 'father' and consequently client roles are created and negotiated during professional meetings. While knowledge is perceived both as pre-understandings or internalised conceptions as well as something constituted in interaction and in professional narratives (Taylor and White, 2000, pp 43-4), knowledge in use rather than the restricted categories was explored.

Ambiguity expressed and demonstrated by a mother was recognisable in the reflections of one of the social workers:

> "When she explains herself, I think she is verbally rather powerful, and expresses her own insight as she quotes: 'Nobody knows better than me and nobody may admit more fully than me, that things have been difficult and that I may have problems' – however, I think that what is lacking, is that this insight is fluctuating, and occasionally she has no insight at all." (Social worker)

During the interview, the social worker gave an extensive picture of the mother, and expressed details from the interaction with her as well as her own interpretations. No fixed category directs what kind of action and services are required. The outspoken mother, her reflections on her own past as well as her efforts to change her life, give the social worker multiple messages. The mother asks for help, but rejects the suggestion that there is reason for concern about her care for the children. Ambiguity and doubt construct the plot in the social worker's narrative:

> "I think that we occasionally engage an expert just to confirm that things are ok.... But in this case I think it is a good idea to bring in an expert [a psychologist], because we don't know enough, and we are not quite certain about our position and I think I would say, I don't feel I have enough knowledge. Sometimes I think I know more than needed, but not in this family. I have not followed the family over an extended period, I have not met the mother sufficiently frequently to see her fluctuations, and I have not met the children, I have not observed the interaction between the mother and the children. If I had done that in a structured way, I believe I could have commented adequately...." (Social worker)

The social worker's knowledge construction is influenced by the mother's ambiguity and her reflections illuminate the interrelated connection of professional sense making and experience. Her uncertainty directs her to search for knowledge that is more reliable, although her knowledge construction principally has a narrative reflective structure. These reflections echo Parton (2000), who claims that uncertainty, complexity and doubt are continuously present in professional social work practice and thus social work expertise cannot be reduced to application of external theories, empirically tested methods or legislation (Hall et al, 2003). Nevertheless, theory is fundamental in creating and negotiating clienthoods and thus professional identity.

In another example, the social worker monitors a mother in her development, emphasizing changes in her attitude and conversation. She says that she and an experienced colleague applied for funding to implement a network-oriented approach in order to strengthen the parenting skills in the family. The family was invited to a course together with another family in a hotel where they received a delicate lunch, something very different from the family's daily life:

> "… it was quite exciting. Because in that situation, we were considering the basics, why we play with children, what level of development their son had reached. You know, the basics, but difficult, too, particularly talking so much about it. Being an ordinary parent, you just do the things that appear right to you. You do not think about the basic psychological principles, but we did talk about them in a way, and then we talked about the parents' childhood." (Social worker)

In this study, the interaction process between the social workers and families and the professional positions were significant factors in construction of conspicuous normative knowledge as well as discursive reflecting knowledge. Knowledge in use was indirectly identified through narrative analysis and analysis of narratives (Polkinghorne, 1995). The position of the social workers and construction of professional identity is thus a result of interactive work with individuals and families. Moreover, clients and clienthoods are constructed and developed in interactive processes.

In an ongoing English study involving semi-structured interviews with social workers and managers, participants are asked to discuss and analyse what they understand by 'evidence-based practice' and to illustrate how this understanding may affect their work with clients. Results suggest that for some practitioners, like the Norwegian staff in the study described earlier, what is considered to be most useful knowledge can be interpreted as having a narrative structure; however more formal research or 'evidence-based' knowledge is also useful, yet it is different (the value of more formal knowledge tended in this study to be expressed more directly by managers). One social worker illustrates how, in his dealings with clients, his professional reactions could be quite individualised:

> "I think that sometimes strengths and also weaknesses of social work is that we're never going to agree on what social work is about, what its role is in society. And so it is going to be contested, so it's different for me, from the person who sits next to me in this team. And our way of doing it is going to be different, and then I think the thresholds of when it's right that the state will intervene with a family and say right, we are going to get involved with your family are going to be different from different members of the same [social work] team." (Social worker)

This example also illustrates that the worker recognises that many ambiguities are embedded in social work, but he tries to use these rather than always seeing them as a disadvantage professionally. In particular he focuses on a key theory or model of 'relationship-based practice' bringing him closer to clients (as opposed to 'therapeutic' theories or approaches he learnt at college). We suggest that this also relates to a 'narrative' understanding of processes involved with direct practice:

> "I've only been practicing for three and half years in social work, but I think from college social work ... I think there was more emphasis on that perhaps therapeutic aspect of social work. Although there's a more recent kind of model of theory about good 'relationship-based' social work, which really kind of appeals to me, because I like that bit about the best work comes from forming a relationship with the parent, the child...."

In comparison, this worker describes a 'managerial' approach that would imply greater reliance on research 'evidence', suggesting more standardised responses to clients. This comparison indicates that development of professional identity can be a contextual struggle. As we shall see, it begins during and continues after education and requires continued analytical reflection.

Analytical reflection: a contextual struggle

Bell and Villadsen's work (2011) demonstrates how English social work students and their social work educators (tutors) viewed knowledge and the support given to students via 'tutor groups'; these are intended to enable them to reflect and build up acceptable social work identities over the whole of their professional education and beyond.[1] Qualitative project data reveal issues relating to perceived 'acceptable' social work values and practices, and suggest how these could be used by student social workers over time as professional identity/ies developed. Both tutors and students recognised the support and monitoring functions of tutor groups; however, students emphasised their supportive function while staff highlighted monitoring of student progression and development, and fitness for practice. Tutors were well aware of organisational factors outside the university that, over time, would continually affect development of student social workers' identities, both positively and negatively:

> "… there's a bit of a dilemma for us, I think, sometimes because we have to give a balanced view of practice. You know, we maybe sometimes give a rose-tinted view of what social work's about. Then they go out there and they find the reality is different; they've got to work with teams. Whereas sometimes the core value base of social work, social justice, anti-discriminatory practice is not always reflected in the organisation. And there are politics and there are issues about them being students, so issues of power. So I think a core aspect of our work is actually enabling them manage being in a practice context." (Tutor)

Students involved in this English study suggested the tutor group was a 'safe haven' for them that, during their studies, enabled them to deal with 'practice' influences and to build up a more realistic professional identity:

> "I think there are common themes that emerge in a group, so I think when you're in [work] placement you're isolated and you're all on your own and when you come back to your group you realise other people are going through the same thing." (Student)

The tutor's role in enabling these English social work students to develop their professional identities was crucial, not least because the tutor may have had many years of practical social work experience:

> "And it's also good to get the tutor's point of view because it's good to get their knowledge and understanding. And our tutor, like many of them, has quite a number of years of experience. And it's always quite good for the tutor to reflect and to tell us about things, issues that they've been through, so I find it really helpful." (Student)

In effect, the 'tutor groups' that were examined in this study were acting as a mediating and 'liminal' space (Czarniawska and Mazza, 2003) where students and tutors could reflect 'inwards' about the educational setting and knowledge students were receiving and working with in that context, and 'outwards' into social work practice and work with clients. These two 'different worlds' can sometimes link to and represent ideal and actual forms of practice, both being visible to participants within this liminal space. By a process of analytical reflection, tutors and students could support each other to make sense of what was happening to them in daily practice, and suggest how they could construct appropriate identities and professional values.

However, research shows this struggle is not only related to becoming a professional during education. It is also a struggle for recently educated social workers who experience the difference between being a student and a social worker in practice, and, in relation to this, how constructing a professional identity is an endeavour. The Danish social workers refer to their education as underpinning a holistic view of the client, and a professional identity related to helping and supporting people in difficult life situations. The possibility of actually upholding this identity is considered a struggle and largely dependent on the political, economic, organisational and managerial context, as expressed as follows:

> "Many times my manager said: 'We are not to offer the children, [what is for their best], but what is sufficient.' This was the values underpinning our work, and it was completely open and clearly how we should not offer what was considered the best, and I simply couldn't deal with it." (Social worker)"This really surprised me. I thought, I should go out and do some social work. Well, I must say I haven't done that yet." (Social worker)

A major issue among social workers is how they deal with this discrepancy between on the one hand identity constructed through education, on the other experience of acting in professional practice requiring a certain approach to problem solving. Two different approaches are conveyed. Some social workers insist on cultivating professional knowledge including theoretical knowledge. They tend to view professional identity as developed through education: "Our basic knowledge comes from education. It is not something you think of everyday, but if you begin to reflect, this is where it comes from" (Danish social worker). Some social workers also approach learning as based on reflection on different forms of knowledge:

> "A lot of knowledge comes from education and from experience. You get some good theories from education, but sometimes you … when you get out from education and move into reality, it might not be everything which is usable and resembles practice, but in this way you also learn something." (Social worker)

In contrast, other social workers view knowledge and values promoted in education as too 'rosy' or 'idealistic' compared with professional practice governed by political, economic, managerial conditions. They favour a more 'realistic' approach in education, and argue that this will strengthen professional identity: "At least I have experienced some colleagues, who have suffered a breakdown, because they feel it is impossible to do the kind of social work they really want to do … this is not how reality is" (social worker).

These Danish social workers emphasise the need for more 'practice-oriented' education and to learn something that is usable and directly applicable in practice. They have experienced a 'cultural shock' and feel positioned in between 'two different worlds':

> "I remember when I was a trainee. We thought the social workers were outlaws, totally stressed and couldn't think one theoretical thought anymore, and I still think like that, but now I also feel, how it disappears more and more…." (Social worker)

Different approaches among social workers stem from *both* the experience of acting in practice *and* from an analytical reflection on relations between different forms of knowledge as they are beginning to construct a professional identity. Within this process translating and recombining different forms of knowledge into a professional identity is at stake. All the social workers in our Danish and English examples tend to speak of education as something different from 'reality' and of practice as something 'outside' education. In the process of constructing a professional identity, they are highly orientated towards practice and being competent at solving 'real' problems. But they differ in terms of how they analytically manage to translate and recombine different forms of knowledge. One could argue this is exactly because they are recently educated. However, construction of a professional identity is a lifelong process, which requires time.[2]

Time: an unnoticed constituent of professional identity?

Experiences as well as analytical reflection are constructs based in and taking place over time, although the significance of time in these contexts may often be unnoticed. We have already described how English students needed time to assimilate their practical experiences of social work, reflecting on these in relation to ideas about 'evidence-based practice' in the presence of tutors who had already had many years of practical experience and theoretical knowledge. This enabled students to approach the process of building their identities analytically as well as through building personal reflective narratives.

In interviews with Danish social work managers, with years of social work experience but recently participating in a Master's programme, there are several examples of how the process of developing professional identity involves experience as well as analytical reflection on the relation between various forms of knowledge. These Master's students are primarily orientated towards learning that can benefit the development of professional identities, knowledge, values and practices at their workplace. However, these students convey how this is only possible if they strengthen their competences to conduct and promote analytical reflection in particular about the relation between theory and practice. This is the main reason why they return to education on a higher level. All the social work managers emphasise how they use analytical reflection on various forms of knowledge to develop professional identities in practice – primarily by addressing knowledge in practice:

> "I did an analysis of six cases concerning some of the children with a psychiatric diagnosis. It was a wondering about, what is it about all these diagnoses? Why do they keep on getting these diagnoses? One of the things I found out was that we are actually asking for them ourselves, mainly because it is difficult to help these children. And in addition to this, we were actually not using theory qualified or thoroughly enough to be able to understand the needs of the child. There is so much, not common sense, but practical experiences at play in this work." (Social work manager)

One should not mistakenly assume that what is promoted is analytical reflection that neglects experiential aspects of professional identity. Construction of professional identity is viewed as a complex process involving 'building up' capacity for reflection in practice:

> "I think, a competent employee, a competent social worker, you have to build her up. She must be trained in thinking and reflection and must be placed in situations where: 'Aha, I have to go back to this, and I have to reflect on this again.' A manager must be able to ask interesting questions. A manager must also be able to show, I have some doubts on

> this too. Make sure that professionals are met with questions instead of answers, so that their ability to reflect is trained." (Social work manager)

This process of 'building' professional identity is considered an important task. It is also considered as a way of promoting professional identity in wider organisational, managerial, economic and political contexts. As an example, some social work managers critically reflected on expectations for documentation, standardisation and evidence based practice. They emphasised how professionals should become 'knowledgeable', sustaining a 'sensitive' as well as an analytical approach to lived experiences of people. This is also inherent in their reflections on their own development:

> "Well, I have a lot of knowledge based on my experience. But actually, it is a bit difficult to point out, where did it come from? Maybe, it is because I translate a lot of knowledge, which has then become my experience, which I haven't thought of as knowledge I have." (Social work manager)

These examples illustrate how development of professional identity is a lifelong process dependent on both experiential and more abstract forms of knowledge. This double reference requires analytical reflection. It is a question of whether the current environment for developing professional practice in social work sufficiently underpins this. In particular, is it recognised that developing professional identity requires time?

Conclusion

In this chapter we have attempted to explore some processes involved in professional identity construction in social work, going across the continuum of professional education and everyday practice. We have seen from our examples that experience, analytical reflection and time can allow identities to be 'built' gradually; the sometimes oppositional perspectives of 'ideal' versus 'actual' underpin different types of knowledge (theoretical/practical) and educational and practice 'worlds' encountered by students, tutors and practitioners. We suggest that space for analytical reflection is crucial in mediating professionals' understandings of their practice, revealing how their own identities are being constructed. In some cases an actual 'liminal' space such as a 'tutor group' or possibilities for 'lifelong education', neither solely in a practice nor an educational context, can help participants to progress their own professional development. At other times these accomplishments are achieved by direct practice and reflection about those practices.

Having explored and demonstrated how building professional identity, involving the development of a set of beliefs, attitudes and understanding, is related to complex processes of construction, it becomes clear that promoting a professional identity is not simply related to the use of 'evidence-based' or other research-based sources of knowledge. This is not to say that such sources of knowledge cannot be used in, and inform certain aspects of, practice. However, as we have tried to demonstrate, construction of professional identity requires experience, analytical reflection and time. This is not something that comes 'automatically' from using research-based knowledge seen as 'evidence'. Instead it is a lifelong process of learning, acting and reflecting in education and practice. If one believes in an 'evidence base' focused on research as the 'key' to building professional identities and competencies 'effectively' and fast, one tends to overlook how construction of professional identity requires time and space – time for obtaining experience, time for constructing a set of beliefs, attitudes and understandings, and time for analytical reflection. The latter is above all crucial in enabling professionals to be continuously aware of and to survey the power as well as a self-interest embedded in all professions and professional positions.

Notes

1 This project involved semi-structured interviews with a group of 11 social work educators, focus groups with students and detailed observation of tutor-facilitated student seminars ('tutor groups') in England. I acknowledge the support of all participants and my co-researcher Aase Villadsen.

2 This example derives from an analysis of 11 interviews with social work managers included in a Danish Master's programme (Nissen, 2013). The interviews and the analysis were part of a larger interview study and research project conducted at Aalborg University as part of the masters' programme on Vulnerable Children and Young People (Kildedal et al, 2013).

References

Argyris, C. and Schön, D.A. (1996) *Organizational learning II: Theory, method, and practice*, Reading, MA: Addison-Wesley.

Barth, F. (2000) 'Boundaries and connections', in A.P. Cohen (ed) *Signifying identities: Anthropological perspectives on boundaries and contested values*, London: Routledge.

Bell, L. (2015) 'Ethics, values and social work identity(ies)', in L. Bell and T. Hafford-Letchfield (eds) *Ethics and values in social work practice*, Maidenhead, Berkshire: McGraw-Hill/ Open University Press.

Bell, L. and Villadsen, A. (2011) '"A sense of belonging": examining how social work students acquire professional values, identities and practice competence through group support', Paper presented at 1st European Social Work Research Conference, St Catherine's College, Oxford University, March.

Czarniawska, B. and Mazza, C. (2003) 'Consulting as a liminal space', *Human Relations*, 56(3): 267-90.

Dreyfus, H.L. and Dreyfus, S.E. (1986) *Mind over machine*, New York, NY: Basic Books.

Gilgun, J.E. (2005) 'The four cornerstones of evidence-based practice in social work', *Research on Social Work Practice*, 15(1): 52-61.

Gobet, F. and Chassy, P. (2009) 'Expertise and intuition: a tale of three theories', *Minds and Machines*, 19(2): 151-80.

Hall, C., Juhila, K., Parton, N. and Pösö, T. (2003) *Constructing clienthood in social work and human services: Interaction, identities, and practices*, London: Jessica Kingsley.

Jenkins, R. (2004) *Social identity*, Oxford and New York, NY: Routledge.

Kildedal, K., Laursen, E. and Michelsen, M. (eds) (2013) *Socialfaglig ledelse. Børne- og Ungeområdet* [Social Work Management. Social Services for Children and Young People], Copenhagen: Samfundslitteratu.

Nissen, M.A. (2010) *Nye horisonter i socialt arbejde - En refleksionsteori* [New horizons in social work - A reflection theory], Copenhagen: Akademisk Forlag.

Nissen, M.A. (2013) *Lederen som udforsker af socialfagligt myndighedsarbejde – vidensformer og kompetencer* [The manager as an explorer of social case work – forms of knowledge and kompentences], in K. Kildedal, E. Laursen and M. Michelsen (eds) *Socialfaglig ledelse. Børne- og Ungeområdet* [Social Work Management. Social Services for Children and Young People], Copenhagen: Samfundslitteratur, pp 161-77.

Nissen, M.A. and Harder, M. (2009) 'Changes in social welfare – on the experience of governance and the strategies of social workers', *Nordisk Sosialt Arbeid*, 3/4: 233-45 (published in Danish).

Nissen, M.A., Harder, M. and Andersen, M.B. (2008) *Socialrådgiverenes fremtidige kvalifikation og og kompetencer* [The future qualifications and competences of social workers], Aalborg: Aalborg University.

Oettingen, von A. (2007) 'Pedagogical theories of action in the difference between theory and practice', in A. von Oettingen and F. Wiedemann (eds) *Between theory and practice – Contemporary challenges for pedagogical and professional education*, Odense: University Press of South Denmark, pp 17-52 (published in Danish).

Parton, N. (2000) 'Some thoughts on the relationship between theory and practice in and for social work', *British Journal of Social Work*, 30(4): 449-63.

Polkinghorne, D.E. (1995) 'Narrative configuration in qualitative analysis', *Qualitative Studies in Education*, 8(1): 5-23.

Robinson, W.P. (ed) (1996) *Social groups and identities: Developing the theory of Henri Tajfel*, London: Butterworth Heinemann.

Schön, D.A. (1983) *The reflective practitioner: How professionals think in action*, New York, NY: Basic Books.

Taylor, C. and White, S. (2000) *Practising reflexivity in health and welfare: Making knowledge*, Buckingham: Open University Press.

Trede, F., Macklin, R. and Bridges, D. (2012) 'Professional identity development: a review of the higher education literature', *Studies in Higher Education*, 37(3): 365-84.

Vindegg, J. (2011) 'Å forstå en familie. Fortellinger som kunnskapskilde i sosialarbeideres profesjonelle yrkesutøvelse' [Understanding a family. Narratives as a source of knowledge in social workers' professional practice], PhD thesis, Oslo: Høgskolen i Oslo.

Webb, S.A. (2001) 'Some considerations on the validity of evidence-based practice in social work', *British Journal of Social Work*, 31(1): 57-79.

FOUR

Professional supervision and professional autonomy

Synnöve Karvinen-Niinikoski, Liz Beddoe, Gillian Ruch and Ming-sum Tsui

Introduction

Through professional supervision, practitioners engage in a relationship with a supervisor enabling both a place and space to refine and develop professional identity, knowledge and skills and for reflectively examining the challenges faced in everyday practice. Supervision itself has a long history and is a well-established component of the health and social care professions. In recent years, however, relentless changes in the nature of professional roles within these contexts have led to corresponding variations in how professional practice supervision is configured and delivered (Karvinen-Niinikoski, 2009). As a contested practice, the linking of supervision and managerial surveillance in social work is not new (Beddoe, 2010); this tension is also considered in Karvinen-Niinikoski's (2004) discussion on critical reflection and supervision.

These challenges are increasingly associated with the dominance of New Public Management (NPM) practices and their influence on the management of social work services (Beddoe et al, 2015). Manthorpe and colleagues (2013, p 3) note the presence of a kind of dyadic approach in discussions of supervision in social work, where supervision is grasped either as largely introspective (a therapeutic model) or as its antithesis, an instrumental tool for surveillance and the soft exercise of power and authority. Autonomous professionals are presented as reflective professionals with demands for reflexivity in their agency and for relational expertise. In social work they report work stress associated with feelings of losing their professional autonomy and commonly experience a sense of management intrusion into clinical decision making (Lymbery, 1998). With the advent of new models of public management, and technologies of control such as evidence-based practice and clinical governance, managerial bureaucracies are asserting greater control of the professions than ever (Coburn, 2006). In response to these changes the expansion of supervision can be understood as a likely forum for the maintenance and development of unique professional expertise.

Tensions between professional autonomy and managerial accountability are also reflected in the changing positions of professions more broadly (Tsui and Cheung, 2004). The links between NPM and professionalism in the public service context of western post-industrial societies has been examined by Evetts (2009). Evetts was interested in clarifying to what extent a new and different type of professionalism is developing and depicts an emerging mixture of two ideal types of professions: the organisational and the occupational. The first type is manifested in a discourse of control used increasingly by managers in workplaces. The latter is based on practitioner autonomy, discretionary judgment and assessment, particularly in complex cases, and resonates with perceptions of supervision in social work settings.

Concerns about professional autonomy are widely expressed by professionals and researchers in the welfare professions. Within the field of social work, this is a constant issue arguably connected to the expansion of NPM in neoliberal regimes and the reconfigurations of welfare services associated with it. For social workers in particular, anxieties about professional autonomy appear to be particularly salient and associated with a fear of professional freedom being constrained in the face of the controlling nature of NPM practices and attendant bureaucracy. In turn, this can be experienced as an undermining of the profession's basic values. This call for professional autonomy seems relentless and imbued with a deterministic resignation. It is also suggested that processes that have become visible in sociological studies on welfare professions (for example, Evans, 2010) that acknowledge that the position of professionals is being changed within the organisational rearrangement of welfare services are also a reality for social work professionals.

Within this climate of anxiety, the safeguarding of professional autonomy, expertise and identity (Evans and Harris, 2004) becomes a significant agenda item for professionalisation interests and projects. In this respect, for many professions supervision has been an important medium for strengthening professional identity, identifying coping strategies for personal survival and growth and facilitating the utilisation and transfer of knowledge, as well as being a guarantee of professional quality and credibility. Negotiating new positions within this changing professional context with its new power structures and service demands is not easy but it does raise the question of how a somewhat defeatist cry for professional autonomy could evolve into a more empowering approach. One alternative, within the social work profession, is found in efforts to strengthen professional autonomy through professional supervision and, in doing so, securing both the quality of professional work and the wellbeing of practitioners.

In this chapter we examine how professional supervision and its future are seen by an international group of experts in social work supervision. The aim is to explore evolving perceptions of social work supervision's role, and to what extent these reflections relate to professional autonomy as a central feature of the developmental tensions discussed earlier. The topic has a background in the authors' shared interest in exploring supervision research on an international scale. For this purpose, a Delphi study was conducted over 2013-15 to establish an international dialogue about the visions and prospects of social work supervision and its scholarship and research (Beddoe et al, 2014). The study posed questions on topics such as what social work supervision would look like in 10 years' time and which aspects of it are most worthy of scholarly research. Drawing on data from the Delphi survey and an emerging meta-theoretical understanding of professional supervision as a vehicle for promoting critical professional agency, we discuss some tensions found in the material in relation to professional supervision and development. These dyadic, even circular, reflections reflect how professionals position themselves in changing contexts and the extent to which they experience workplace constraints as threats to their work. Placing supervision in a frame of theoretical understanding of human agency (Emirbayer and Mische, 1998; Eteläpelto et al, 2013) and thus opening a meta-theoretical understanding of supervision, could help the profession undergo significant transformation while remaining subjects of their own expertise.

Central concepts: autonomy, discretion, agency and supervision

The concepts of professional autonomy and supervision are intertwined with a further two topical, and inextricably interconnected, concepts: professional agency and discretion.

Professional autonomy

Professional autonomy (Brante, 2011) is a concept emerging from the professionalisation processes within modern society and theories of professions and professional power (Abbott, 1988). The field of the professions is, according to Abbott, a place of continuous struggle for professional jurisdiction: the owning of the expertise in a particular realm of service. Other theorists of the professions emphasise the safeguarding of professional power with professional autonomy as one central feature (Freidson, 2001). Autonomy is a core concept for classical professionalisation theories (Abbott, 1988) and might be the most salient issue for any profession. Following Abbott's theory, owning this autonomous professional status can be seen as competing for professional and societal power and for legitimacy and jurisdiction of field expertise. The salience of autonomy could also be read as professional freedom that is particularly susceptible to collapse with the expansion of controlling NPM policies and their attendant bureaucratic rules (Evetts, 2009; Evans, 2013).

In the face of rapid structural, societal and political change and shifting epistemological understandings and knowledge policies, professional monopolies have been challenged (Knorr-Cetina, 2007). Consequently, for some decades, the traditional pillars of professional power systems – expertise (knowledge and know-how), institutions (socio-legal structures for exercising expertise) and professional status (power over expertise) – have been progressively undermined and weakened, and professional autonomy is experienced as being under threat (Evetts, 2009; Chandler et al, in Chapter Five of this volume) in many professions, including social work. These threatening processes are identified in neoliberal systems of governance and NPM practices that build on new kinds of control, direction and power systems involving process models and standardisation, invariably based on computerised systems and accountability regimes. Here health and social care professionals face new challenges and risk a diminution of their autonomy. What remains, conceptually, from this loss is today often discussed as professional discretion (Evans, 2010).

Professional discretion

Professional discretion (Evans, 2010, 2013) refers to the relationship between professional agency and organisational rules and to the tension between policy and day-to-day professional practice as a key question in policy and practice. This, in turn, causes problems for professional ethics and, of course, for professional autonomy (Karvinen-Niinikoski, 2009). The concept stems from Lipsky's classical work on 'street-level bureaucracy' (1980), which states that policy implementation in the end comes down to the people who actually implement it – an issue that immediately resonates with understandings of supervision, professional autonomy and agency. Professional discretion is also a concept that challenges the professional cry for the lost autonomy of the professional subject. It resists the configuration of professionals as simply the passive recipients of instructions and structural restrictions and seeks to position them as individuals who possess transformative and responsible professional agency.

Professional agency

Agency, in the context of concerns regarding professional autonomy, can be understood as a mediating concept situated between professional discretion and freedom and the contextual and organisational control contributing to a loss of autonomy and even threatening the core values of professional social work. Agency is also a core concept when discussing critical reflection, professional identity and the subjective position of professionals and, in this sense, it stands as a central concept for theories of supervision. Professional agency is strongly associated with critical reflection and thus lies at the heart of discourses on supervision, adult and professional learning (Karvinen-Niinikoski, 2009; Eteläpelto et al, 2013).

According to Eteläpelto et al (2013), since the 1970s, or alternatively, from 2000 and Mezirow's and Freire's critical pedagogy, Giddens' structuration theory and Archer's critical realism, there has been a growing interest in agency in various scientific fields. The combination of agency and personal identity has continued through feminist post-structuralism into socio-cultural approaches, such as the theory of expansive learning and understandings of the subject positioning of individual agency. By analysing these conceptual developments and drawing from their empirical research Eteläpelto and colleagues (2013, p 62) sum up a subject-centred, socio-cultural approach to professional agency. They conclude that professional agency means that vocational subjects and/or communities are entitled to make choices and use their discretion in ways that affect their work and/or professional identity. Through their personal and professional capacities individuals hold certain agentic resources and engage discursively with all these factors, maintaining temporal connections from the past through to the future.

Rediscovered in discourses on coping with the pressures of diminishing autonomy, for example in social work under the NPM regimes (Kam, 2014), professional agency can be considered as a core concept in recapturing the concept of professional autonomy and connects closely with the concept of professional discretion (Evans, 2010; Eteläpelto et al, 2013). Professional contexts' agency can arguably be seen as an achievement/aim, in which both discretion and the dynamic challenges of working life are met in processes of regeneration and transformation. Control and understanding of professional agency, however, is complicated and raises tensions between practitioners and management (Beddoe, 2010). This has been reflected in the concerns of Nordic social work professionals and academics experiencing continuous restriction of jurisdiction and professional autonomy (Røysum, 2010). In Evetts' (2009) analysis of the managerial confusion and tension governing the two emerging ideal types of professionalism (organisational and occupational), it could be suggested that the primary concern focuses on agency (that is, on being an active societal actor) and its constraints on professionals. Thus the link between autonomy and agency becomes central for supervision, which, in NPM regimes, is also regarded as a sophisticated tool for governance and control.

Agency and discretion are complex concepts, pivotal to the efforts of supervision to help social workers understand their own agency as reflexive professionals in challenging working conditions in a complex society. Agency and its link to the expression of professional identities can also be seen as a central element in theoretical understandings of supervision, in reaching a meta-theoretical understanding of the functional mechanisms of supervision.

Professional supervision

As an essential part of professional and occupational practice, supervision is a key factor in the promotion of practice excellence, productivity and practitioner retention (Koivu, 2013). In emotionally demanding human professions like social work, supervision can provide a necessary containment of emotional relationships and pressures and thus may also perform occupational health functions (Adamson, 2012). In social work, a contested profession from the outset (Houston, 2002), supervision has a long tradition as a process employed to safeguard professional autonomy and expertise and, further, to resist threats to its professional jurisdiction (Tsui, 2005). The centrality of professional and personal growth to the classical aim of supervision is founded on the theoretically grounded ideas of continuous professional development, as well as on more or less hidden ideas of safeguarding professional autonomy (Tsui, 2005). Concerns about protecting professional autonomy are manifest in the Nordic context by a strong emphasis on ensuring that the supervisor is external to the employing welfare service organisation (Karvinen-Niinikoski and Salonen, 2005).

Traditionally supervision has focused on promoting high-quality professional services by supporting the learning, management and development of professional practice among individuals and groups of practitioners in human services professions. An expansion of professional or 'clinical supervision' (Koivu, 2013) has stemmed from recent research on work-related wellbeing and transformative leadership that emphasises the importance of employee engagement in a participative ethos for fostering innovative potential and promoting productivity (Yliruka and Karvinen-Niinikoski, 2013).

Human services work is considered to be emotionally burdening and cognitively challenging because professional values are an essential part of professional expertise providing legitimacy and justification for the professional field in question. In daily practice these values and interests are blurred and require, for clarity, reflective practice. Supervision has traditionally provided a mechanism for promoting professional reflection and enhancing the quality of services. In recent decades the 'preoccupation with … systems of accountability' can be attributed in large part to the 'critique of professional practice' and a 'crisis of trust in professionals' (Davys and Beddoe, 2010, pp 13-14). This 'crisis', according to Evetts (2009, pp 258-62), is a major factor behind changes to professionalising processes and the associated tensions. Within this climate of anxiety about trustworthiness, the safeguarding of professional autonomy, expertise and identity (Evans and Harris, 2004) has become significant for professional projects.

Circular reflections and concerns about professional autonomy and supervision

Our interest in discussing the relationship between professional autonomy and supervision was roused by often-reported concerns about threats to professional autonomy and worsening working conditions in social work, expressed both in research and professional debates in social work and supervision. The concerns found in the literature (Beddoe et al, 2015) informed the design of the Delphi survey, which sought to obtain internationally comparative knowledge about contemporary understandings of social work supervision and perceptions of research gaps in this domain. Our aim in the first phase of the Delphi study on supervision (Beddoe et al, 2015) was to learn about expert opinions and visions about the present state of social work supervision and to gain experts' ideas about the focus of future supervision research.

This study, conducted from 2013-15, was designed as a multi-phase project involving the delivery of two open-ended questionnaires to experts and important stakeholders, such as those with academic expertise in supervision and those whom we might define as 'expert users', for example, individuals involved in supervision as expert practitioners, practice teachers, trainers and those who might be influential in developing and implementing supervision policies within social service organisations. In the replies to this survey reflections were offered by 53 participants from five continents and 15 countries, providing a generous data set, albeit somewhat skewed towards Anglophone countries. Delphi sampling is not intended to be representative but is a means for recruiting knowledgeable, committed participants into a process that pools ideas and creates potential for sophisticated reflection. The analysis of the challenges facing the practice of social work supervision was conducted via thematic coding. Organisational and political factors loomed large as significant influences on how supervision was (or was not) promoted and supported. The impact of service budget cuts under recessionary government policies were also frequently mentioned, along with the impact of a pervasive risk-averse climate (Beddoe et al, 2015).

A somewhat surprising feature of the Delphi study results was how strongly and critically respondents expressed their concerns about the loss of, and threats to, professional discretion and autonomy in social work supervision. These concerns stretched beyond simply threats to professional identity and encompassed fear of the demise of professional supervision as a forum for critical reflection and a site for discussing social work practice-related ethical matters. Reflections illuminating these concerns emerged in response to future focused questions on social work supervision and its significance in practice governance. The answers to these reflected themes around autonomy and proved to be quite circular, drawing both on expressions of the role of supervision in promoting professional strength and fear of supervision becoming a forum for losing power.

One participant captures this circularity: "I fear it's a circular debate and we might be in the same space again and again." Behind this circularity sits tension and uncertainty about how supervision will be used: for "management/competence or reflective learning" or to enhance a "strong but diverse profession mandated to be registered and well educated, critical and expansive thinkers and experimenters.... A group that is bold and able ... creative, experimental ... and radiating hope and innovation...", instead of leaving the profession to stay as "a divided non-professional group who has subsumed or gone beyond social control and re-apportioning dwindling resources". These alternatives reflect social work preoccupations with social justice and the dispositions needed to meet the challenges social workers "face in societies in a local, regional and global sense of the work". These are, in many senses, the core values attached to professional autonomy in social work, and perceived as under threat.

Supervision is also described in optimistic terms, one participant hoping that "social work supervision would be recognised as an important social work practice domain", benefiting both "clients and supervisees". It is also advocated that "social work supervision is conducted more rigorously, making use of what we know works for staff, service users and organisations from the evidence base". There is also a hope that there will be "the momentum towards reflective practice" that would mean "that reflective supervision is highly valued and prioritised within the provision of social work services". Most optimistically this was expressed as follows: "The profile of social work supervision is developing. I would like to see it develop further. Supervision and reflection are essential to the ongoing existence of social work practice in this sense. It is the space away from pressures of practice and mechanistic culture that has developed in the last 30 years." Most important, however, is being supported and valued for coping with the demanding and difficult work: "[s]ocial workers need support to resist and creatively challenge the neoliberal intensification of blaming the person, family or community for things the economic systems produce" and "[s]upervision must encompass the ability to look beyond the individual and connect the dots to systemic cause and effect ... basically social work supervision mirrors and supports social work practice".

When asked about the future, many participants seemed rather resigned: "If nothing is done intentionally, supervision could become nothing more than a tool for administrative surveillance." It is seen to be "pretty well the same – it is not the political climate for much change"; or "more pressed for time; poorer quality" with no improvement; or "not prioritised – worse"; or "Sadly, I do not think there will be a significant shift." The worsening visions are placed "in the context of social welfare organisations due to increasing concern about management, quantitative output and manpower cut[s]". Similar concerns could be discerned 'between the lines' when asked about the most important and urgent questions for research in supervision. There is an interest in refocusing "the practice and discipline value of supervision, understanding that balancing administrative needs will continue to be an ongoing challenge ... [for example] How do supervisors use their power so that social workers' knowledge and skills are valued and developed?" Parallel to seeing supervision as support to professional autonomy, there is the concern about the risk to professional agency and autonomy of having a supervisor as an outsider to one's own profession (Hojer and Bradley, 2009; Beddoe and Howard, 2012). For example, one participant commented: "[I am] not clear how increased regulation will address the need for competent supervision, especially when many other disciplines are represented in the ranks of supervisors."

The reason for this resignation, hesitation and sadness seems to reflect a loss of professional self-determination and autonomy. For one informant this involved supervision aligning itself with neoliberalistic trends and narrower definitions of social work and supervision: "I fear that social work's push for professionalism and accreditation in supervision and practice … is unintentionally dove tailing with, and supporting neo-liberal, managerial, consumerist influences that continue to narrow, shape, re-define what seem reasonable of possible within social work and social work supervision.… I fear that as social workers we are contributing to devaluing the core of our work." A particularly gloomy vision was that "at worst a divided non-professionalised group who have been subsumed or persuaded by politics of individual blame shame and greed and are unable to go beyond social control and re-apportioning dwindling resources on a 'deserving' qualifying criteria that keeps people in boxes and places of non-participation and disenfranchisement".

One is left pondering how circular the argumentation is, repeating the risks of losing autonomy and hoping for professional supervision to have the strength to build support for sound social work practice.

Discussion: how to cross the circular cycles of professional concerns

The narrative of perceived challenges to professional autonomy alongside hopes for improving the positioning of the profession via the future development of supervision that emerge from this study suggests that the concept of supervision is understood and indeed utilised in many different ways in various contexts (Beddoe, 2015). Alluding to this issue of context and location in approaches to supervision, a research participant commented that "supervision in social work needs to engage with local and global knowledge to assist social workers wherever they are to maintain their focus on meeting the practical and emotional needs of the individuals, families and communities they serve, in an economic climate where this is increasingly difficult".

The cycle of threats and hopes regarding professional autonomy and values-based social work practice suggests ambiguous responses to changing realities. This is understandable, given the trends, described by Evetts (2009), towards the organisational and occupational professions having diminishing powers when considering the more positive future visions it is possible to identify a determination to become stronger, regardless of pressures and constraints. This leaves us with a question as to whether the missing and mediating cycle-breaking concept might actually be the professional agency so central to professional identity and professional emancipation.

As posed by Eteläpelto and colleagues (2013), professional agency is a powerful concept dealing with the professional's identity and capability for making choices and using discretional opportunities in ways that affect their work and/or professional identity. This also means disrupting the circular structures and crossing the boundaries of professional discourses, be they singularly profession-centred or multi-professionally relational, as Edwards (2010) has it. Agency is a concept based on careful ontological analyses of the issues and tensions between individual action and structural constraints (Emirbayer and Mische, 1998; Eteläpelto et al, 2013); the dynamics inherent in the research can be construed as practitioners experiencing a loss of professional autonomy.

An understanding of professional agency is needed especially for creatively developing one's own work and working contexts, for learning at work and for negotiating professional identity (Eteläpelto et al, 2013). It is needed in order to see the options for taking professional responsibility and action. The theoretical understanding of agency might help solve the helplessness syndrome of social work expressed in the circular argumentation above. It is very much what one tries to promote when tackling the circular concerns of losing professional autonomy. Understanding one's own agency and its relation to both professional discretion and autonomy might help emancipating social work to cope with the changing professional structures in changing societies (Kam, 2014).

Conclusion

These reflections on supervision and its future raise questions about the logic of a persistent, circular, professional discourse that is creating and perpetuating resigned attitudes around social work. There remains a strong belief, however, in supervision as an emancipatory support for professional self-respect and identity. It is the potential loss of professional autonomy that may be seen as a major tension. This is also seen in the fear of losing supervision as a reflective professional sphere where a genuine social work professional and ethical ethos can be fostered. These tensions and fears appear similar to those factors lying behind the 'tension model of changing professionalisation' presented by Evetts (2009). The same kinds of discussions have been identified also in the late concerns of losing 'the social' from social work (Røysum, 2010) and even the loss of the social itself (Kam, 2014). The tension model also provides a concept with which to analyse and understand human actors' positions and discretional opportunities in professional practice, in between individual and structural factors and constraints, the factors that are considered as opposite poles in the reflections on the future of social work and supervision.

There is also a strong alternative, and theoretically grounded, approach based on the traditions of 'critically reflective supervision' helping to recognise and manage the fine balance between support and surveillance or managerial organisational dimensions. Meta-theoretical understanding of professional supervision in the frame of human agency will help both practitioners and supervisors to construct sustainable and proactive social work. Instead of despairing about the loss of autonomy, the professionals may go through significant societal and professional transformations as subjects of their own expertise and professional agency.

References

Abbott, A. (1988) *The system of professions. An essay on the division of expert labor*, Chicago, IL: University of Chicago Press.

Adamson, C. (2012) 'Supervision is not politically innocent', *Australian Social Work*, 65(2): 185-96, doi:10.1080/0312407x.2011.618544.

Beddoe, L. (2010) 'External supervision in social work: power, space, risk, and the search for safety', *Australian Social Work*, 65(2): 197-213.

Beddoe, L. (2015) 'Supervision and developing the profession: one supervision or many?', *China Journal of Social Work*, 8(2): 150-63.

Beddoe, L. and Howard, F. (2012) 'Interprofessional supervision in social work and psychology: mandates and (inter) professional relationships', *The Clinical Supervisor*, 31(2): 178-202.

Beddoe, L., Karvinen-Niinikoski, S., Ruch, G. and Tsui, M-S. (2015) 'Towards an international consensus on social work supervision: a report on the first phase of a Delphi study', *British Journal of Social Work*, 8(2): 150-63.

Brante, T. (2011) 'Professions as science-based occupations', *Professions & Professionalization*, 1(1): 4-20.

Coburn, D. (2006) 'Medical dominance then and now: a critical reflection', *Health Sociology Review*, 15(5): 432-43.

Davys, A. and Beddoe, L. (2010) *Best practice in professional supervision. A guide for the helping professions*, London: Jessica Kingsley.

Edwards, A. (2010) *Being an expert professional practitioner. The relational turn in expertise*, London: Springer.

Emirbayer, M. and Mische, A. (1998) 'What is agency?', *American Journal of Sociology*, 103(4): 962-1023.

Eteläpelto, A., Vähäsantanen, K., Hökkä, P. and Paloniemi, S. (2013) 'What is professional agency? Conceptualising professional agency at work', *Educational Research Review*, 10: 45-65.

Evans, T. (2010) *Professional discretion in welfare services: Beyond street-level bureaucracy*, Aldershot: Ashgate.

Evans, T. (2013) 'Organisational rules and discretion in adult social work', *British Journal of Social Work*, 43(4): 739-58.

Evans, T. and Harris, J. (2004) 'Street-level bureaucracy, social work and the (exaggerated) death of discretion', *British Journal of Social Work*, 34(6): 871-95.

Evetts, J. (2009) 'New professionalism and New Public Management: changes, continuities and consequences', *Comparative Sociology*, 8(2): 247-66.

Freidson, E. (2001) *Professionalism. The third logic*, Cambridge: Polity Press.

Hojer, S. and Bradley, G. (2009) 'Supervision reviewed: reflections on two different social work models in England and Sweden', *European Journal of Social Work*, 12(1): 71-85.

Houston, S. (2002) 'Reflecting on habitus, field and capital: towards a culturally sensitive social work', *Journal of Social Work*, 2(2): 149-67.

Kam, P.K. (2014) 'Back to the "social" of social work: reviving the social work profession's contribution to the promotion of social justice', *International Social Work*, 57(6): 723-40.

Karvinen-Niinikoski, S. (2004) 'Social work supervision: contributing to innovative knowledge production and open expertise', in N. Gould and M. Baldwin (eds) *Social work, critical reflection and the learning organisation*, Aldershot: Ashgate, pp 23-40.

Karvinen-Niinikoski, S. (2009) 'Promises and pressures of critical reflection for social work coping in change', *European Journal of Social Work*, 12(3): 333-48.

Karvinen-Niinikoski, S. and Salonen, J. (2005) 'Spänningar inom handledningsdiskussionen' [Tensions in discussing supervision], *Nordisk Sosialt Arbeid*, 3.

Knorr-Cetina, K. (2007) 'Culture in global knowledge societies: knowledge cultures and epistemic cultures', *Interdisciplinary Science Reviews*, 32(4): 361-75.

Koivu, A. (2013) 'Clinical supervision and well-being at work: a four year follow-up study on female hospital nurses', Publications of the University of Eastern Finland, Dissertations in Health Sciences, available at http://epublications.uef.fi.

Lipsky, M. (1980) *Street-level bureaucracy: Dilemmas of the individuals in public service*, New York, NY: Russell Sage Foundation.

Lymbery, M. (1998) 'Care management and professional autonomy: the impact of community care legislation on social work with older people', *British Journal of Social Work*, 28(6): 863-78.

Manthorpe, J., Moriarty, J., Hussein, S., Stevens, M. and Sharpe, E. (2013) 'Content and purpose of supervision in social work practice in England: views of newly qualified social workers, managers and directors', *British Journal of Social Work*, 45(1): 52-68.

Røysum, A. (2010) 'Nav-reformen: sosialarbeidernes profesjon utfordres' [The Nav reform: a challenge to professional social work], *Fontene Forskning*, 1: 41-52.

Tsui, M.S. (2005) *Social work supervision: Contexts and concepts*, Thousand Oaks, CA: Sage Publications.

Tsui, M.S. and Cheung F.C.H. (2004) 'Gone with the wind: the impacts of managerialism on human services', *British Journal of Social Work*, 34(3): 437-42.

Yliruka, L. and Karvinen-Niinikoski, S. (2013) 'How can we enhance productivity in social work? Dynamically reflective structures, dialogic leadership and development of transformative expertise', *Journal of Social Work Practice*, 27(2): 191-206.

Part 2
Control, regulation and management

FIVE

Reconfiguring professional autonomy? The case of social work in the UK

John Chandler, Elisabeth Berg, Marion Ellison and Jim Barry

Introduction

The history of social work in the United Kingdom is a long and complex one, and there are no signs of it getting less complex. If the theory and practice of UK social work is of interest to an international audience, it is not just because of the hegemony of the English language, but also because it has often been at the forefront of changes – for good and ill, perhaps. If there is something to learn from the UK experience, it might be as much from the wrong turns and difficulties of the occupation in that divided realm, as from the advances in thinking and practice. This chapter focuses on the contemporary position of social work in the UK, and on the challenges to what is seen as a managerial-technicist version of social work (Harlow, 2003). If the UK is to be seen as at the forefront of the New Public Management and of managerialist reforms in the 1980s, those in other countries and contexts might seek to avoid some of the problems of an 'early adopter'. It will be apparent here, however, that the future course of the social work occupation in the UK is by no means fully charted. At best we can point to certain possibilities and to social imaginaries that may prove to be the basis for revised forms of practice, however liminal these are. In this discussion the focus will be the degree of professional autonomy of social workers as an occupational group as a feature of these possibilities. First, we focus on the situation from the 1990s to the present day in which this managerial-technicist version of social work takes root and flourishes. Second, we focus on three alternatives that have emerged in recent years. In doing so, we do not intend to provide an indication of the likely direction of travel for UK social work, nor do we assume that these alternatives are the only ones available; we hope merely to draw attention to possible alternatives that might be worth considering and supporting.

The 'profession' of social work in the UK can be regarded as occupying a favourable position, in that social work is a protected title and only those who have undergone graduate-level education in social work, in approved courses, can describe themselves as 'social workers'. This means that many occupational groups providing social care, who might, in other countries, be seen as social workers are not so regarded in the UK. This can be seen as a successful case of professionalisation in which the occupational group comes to gain a measure of closure and construct barriers to entry, based on a distinct body of knowledge and expertise, a step that fully confirms its professional status. However, a cursory glance at the literature on social work in the UK will confirm that this is not how members of the occupation or associated academic commentators construe the situation. If the development of social work in the UK has a long history of debates about the status of the occupation, as well as about the organisational structures appropriate for practice and about the knowledge that is appropriately used by practitioners, then this shows no sign of changing: social work in the UK perennially seems to be 'at the crossroads', to borrow from the title of an article by Lymbery (2001). While systems and structures may vary across the various countries of the UK, they have all endured the challenges of a managerial-technicist reconstruction of social work within a New Public Management paradigm. However, there are many roads that could be taken from this point. The purpose of this chapter is to signpost three alternatives to the managerial-technicist form of social work that have emerged in the social work literature in recent. First, though, in the next section, we seek to clarify the context in which these 'alternatives' have emerged.

Reconfiguration 1: social work in managerialist times

The UK is widely recognised as a country at the forefront of the New Public Management. From the 1980s onwards the pace of reform in the public sector was swift. If the New Public Management is regarded as more of a toolbox than a fixed model (Schedler and Proeller, 2002), the key features were seen to include the adoption of private sector styles and forms of management. This included performance management through targets and measures of performance, the disaggregation and decentralisation of services, often including privatisation and marketisation, and a preoccupation with efficiency (see Pollitt, 1990; Hood, 1991). For Clarke and Newman (1997), this implied a change in regimes of power from one based on 'bureau-professionalism' to one of 'managerialism'. A number of writers have associated such reforms with the rise of neoliberalism (Ferguson, 2008; Harlow et al, 2013). In all this, private sector techniques such as cultural re-engineering to win the hearts and minds of reluctant or recalcitrant workforces thought to be in need of inspirational leadership, and performance management to ensure ongoing commitment and to track progress in meeting managerially designed targets or benchmarks, became the order of the day. Social work became embroiled in the 'audit culture' (Power, 1997), with inspection regimes assessing the 'quality' of provision, and with social workers increasingly subject to targets and objectives. Carey (2009) saw such change as nothing less than the proletarianisation of social work as its practitioners increasingly became subject to managerial control and deskilling through the imposition of protocols for diagnosis and intervention. In this process computer-based systems were not a neutral tool but part of the means by which change was brought about. Increasingly the front-line social worker's practice was driven by the demands of the system so that, according to a study by White (2009), 60-80% of social workers' time was taken up with report writing rather than in talking to clients or colleagues. The practice of supervision by fellow professionals was also seen as becoming managerialised, with reflection on cases and learning from experience in conversation with more experienced colleagues increasingly replaced by discussion of means of meeting 'targets' (Carey, 2009).

Of course the extent to which social work can be 'proletarianised' is open to question. The requirement for graduate-level education might indicate some need for higher-level cognitive functioning – of only a partial separation of 'conception' and 'execution'. However, this can also be seen as an attempt to socialise students into ways of thinking and modes of practice that put assessment and auditing at the heart of the process. Moreover, the extent to which such education focuses on techniques that 'work' – on 'evidence-based practice' – might be part of the process of routinising and rationalising practice.

The development of evidence-based practice within social work, generally, can be seen as an integral part of the development of a managerialised social work practice.

In the UK evidence-based practice came to be promoted through organisations such as the Social Care Institute for Excellence (www.scie.org.uk) and Research in Practice (www.rip.org.uk). However, whatever the hopes of proponents of evidence-based practice, national bodies such as SCIE or RIP cannot necessarily expect their ideas to be taken up in a straightforward way by practitioners, even assuming practitioners become aware of them. This is reinforced by the available literature, which sets evidence-based practice and knowledge use by practitioners in the context of managerialism in the public services (see, for example, Evans and Harris, 2004; Aronson and Smith, 2011; Evans, 2011). Gupta and Blewett (2007) have, however, emphasised the way in which managerialism is mediated by practitioners and their managers alike, with resistances, blockages and refusals part of the process (see also Clarke, 2004). The literature on organisations and work is replete with analyses of how workers who are subject to control and management resist such controls or react in ways that managers might not anticipate or favour (Ackroyd and Thompson, 1999). Of course, social workers who find the working situation uncongenial might also adopt another strategy – exit. And there has been much concern about the difficulties of retaining social workers, much of which points to the dissatisfactions of the job as 'push' factors lead to exit and point to the need for reform (Harlow, 2004).

In the following section we look at some of the ways in which social workers and commentators on social work in the UK have attempted to provide alternatives to the managerial-technicist orthodoxy. Three 'alternatives' are presented. The first is based on academic work that points to a reconfiguration of professional practice away from a managerial-technicist conception; the second is a model that was developed in one UK social work organisation and has since been applied elsewhere in the UK (albeit, with local variations); while the third again comes from the literature on social work, rather than being practice-based. Whether these alternatives offer a reconfiguration of the occupation in ways that offer social workers some degree of autonomy is examined.

Reconfiguration 2: beyond managerialism?

Alternative 1: reconfiguring social work through reconfiguring practice

Without wishing to suggest that the demise of managerialism is a reality, alternative voices are in evidence. The call for 'evaluation in practice' (Shaw, 2011) can be seen as an attempt to reinvigorate professionalism in the face of managerialism and more positivist forms of evidence-based practice.

Evaluation can, of course, have managerialist connotations, with auditing, inspection, performance management and accountability all resting on evaluation. Much depends, though, on the nature of the evaluation and who does the evaluation. Shaw (2011, p 44) draws on interviews with social workers to bring out a distinction they make between a more onerous type of evaluation, 'evaluation proper' – which involves scrutiny from above and is formal, time-consuming, relies on quantitative methods and is external to practice concerns and, on the other hand, 'my kind of practice' or what the social worker does in their day-to-day practice that can be seen as 'evaluation in action'; this is more personal, informal and qualitative. Shaw advocates 'evaluation in practice' that is more like the latter. However, he is also looking to change practice and perhaps to elevate it. As he puts it: 'Evaluating in practice challenges social work to new understandings and new methodologies – and it holds the promise of keeping social work honest' (Shaw, 2011, p 1). These are bold claims from a proselytiser. He is not advocating a comfortable, complacent strategy of blinkered practice, resting on established routines and customs – rather he advocates practices of translation, counter-colonising, interrupting and inhabiting (pp 12-13), designed to challenge assumptions and routines. He wants evaluation to pervade practice rather than be additional to it, coming after the event or from outside. He advocates, instead, evaluation being integrated at all stages of practice – assessing, planning, intervening and reviewing (p 21). The ideas and implementation of ideas he presents is complex and open-ended and does not lend itself to a simple statement or description of a model. However, he does list six 'working rules' for practitioners (Shaw, 2011, pp 73-4):

1. Critically reflect on 'our own' practice.
2. Come to know what they know – that is elicit, as far as possible their tacit, personal and cultural knowledge.
3. Begin with the knowledge that service users bring them.
4. Draw on a wide range of sources and methods that are practice relevant – including a wide range of academic disciplines.
5. Draw on team and colleague working.
6. Draw on participatory evaluation with service users.

In such evaluation Shaw advocates the use of autoethnography, ethnography, narrative and life-history methods, focus groups and visual methods. All can be used, he argues, by practitioners in the course of their practice. Practitioners are encouraged to engage with published research (and to contribute to it) but Shaw wants the boundaries between research and practice to be porous, if not eliminated. Moreover, this is not a model of the professional as expert, with the client as passive recipient. Instead the service user is to be listened to, their knowledge and ideas respected and drawn into the evaluation. The evaluation is participatory as well as personal and may involve colleagues, other professionals and service users. While, then, the professional in this model is expected to exercise a high degree of autonomy, it is exercised in negotiation with and in relation to others – it is a kind of relational autonomy (Mackenzie and Stoljar, 2000).

If Shaw points to alternatives to the dominant managerial-technicist view based on a reinvigorated form of professional practice, he is not alone. One attempt to do social work in a different way in the London Borough of Hackney's children's services department has gained a lot of national attention. The protagonists called this 'reclaiming social work' and it is to this we turn next.

Alternative 2: reclaiming social work – type 1

A radical restructuring of social work practice was initiated in the London Borough of Hackney around 2006 in its work with children and families (rather than in adult social care, which was under a different management structure). The changes were led by Goodman and Trowler whose account of the model we rely on here (see Goodman and Trowler, 2012). This has become a prominent example of an attempt to do things differently and has since been emulated elsewhere (Community Care, 2013; Aberdeen City Council, 2014).

As in many change processes, the 'radical' changes advocated by the protagonists in Hackney rested on the denigration of the state of play that preceded it. As Goodman and Trowler put it:

> [Under the old regime] a workforce often incapable of professional, creative and independent thinking had emerged. The profession suffered from a conveyor belt, risk averse mentality to the inevitable detriment of the children and families it sought to serve. As practitioners were further and further removed from any sense of their own responsibility, or capability to effect positive change, or sense of professional pride, a dangerous casualness emerged, where even automated tasks were often done badly.... it was our intention to reclaim social work and change what it had become. (Goodman and Trowler, 2012, p 161)

The key features of the changes implemented in Hackney can be summarised as follows.

First, the model explicitly rests on the '7s' conceptual framework – a model popularised in Peters and Waterman's (1982) best-selling business book of the 1980s that emphasises seven features: strategy, structure, systems, shared values, skills, staff and style. The shared values that Hackney's social work leaders chose to emphasise were those of striving to keep children safely with their families wherever possible, based on social workers intervening in a 'respectful' and 'collaborative' way with families. Procedures were explicitly established as guides, rather than prescriptive routines. Moreover, the strategy included, at its heart, a strategy of recruiting the 'right people' – those with a high level of skill. Initially this was not easy but the leaders of the initiative put in place demanding assessment centre methods to assess verbal reasoning, as well as written assessments and interviews.

At the heart of the Hackney model are small teams or 'units' of five people: the consultant social worker, a social worker, a family therapist or clinical practitioner, a children's practitioner and a unit coordinator. Overall responsibility for a particular case rests with the consultant social worker. The unit coordinator is essentially an administrator – but one who does provide a crucial point of contact for the family and thus is not simply a 'backroom' figure. A key to the model is the effective collaboration of the team in working with the family. Case supervision is via the weekly unit meeting to discuss each case. Proceduralisation is limited, with practitioners encouraged to think through what they want to do and why, and then do it, rather than do it because they are told to: '… any procedure should be brief, instructive and to the point' (Goodman and Trowler, 2012, p 21). Nearly all decisions about the family are made at the level of the team and the most junior members of units have authority to spend money. The style is said to be one that stresses accessibility, where power is used with care and constructively.

> Taking professional responsibility verbally and in writing is a key part of our approach: to own our views and actions and decisions and never to be afraid to change one's mind demonstrating we got it wrong. Doing things differently from the mainstream is not in and of itself problematic, being thoughtful, respectful and intellectually sound in decision-making is most important and should be held in the highest regards. There is no one truth…. For us Reclaiming Social Work holds the future for an effective and highly regarded profession.' (Goodman and Trowler, 2012, p 25).

The approach to practice is described as a systematic approach rooted in the discipline of family and systemic psychotherapy or family therapy. This systemic model has implications for recording what interventions are made, with a clearer family narrative emerging (Goodman and Trowler, 2012, pp 57-68), as well as affecting the interventions themselves, which are examples of relationship-based social work. The model also incorporates the use of Social Learning Theory (SLT) and this is used in professional practice, but in a flexible way. This use of the 'systemic approach' and SLT can be seen as an attempt to reconfigure social work in a way that is both evidence-informed and managed – but as a way of gaining a degree of professional autonomy.

The use of the model was associated with lowering the number of children taken into care and thus reduced expenditure. According to Goodman and Trowler (2012, p 167), it delivered year-on-year efficiency savings. Turnover of staff was also said to be lowered and the use of agency staff reduced. This model does not entail the end of management, but the role of consultant social worker in a unit is said to be very different from that of team manager in the more conventional social work organization. It remains 'rooted in practice', whereas the traditional career structure encouraged progression into non-practitioner roles. This configuration is presented as a less hierarchical, more collaborative model in which the consultant social worker is able to share skills and experience. Above this level, however, is a group manager who deals with more traditional issues associated with the 'line management' of staff. This model, then, does not so much dispense with managerialism as reconfigure it in a less bureaucratic, 'leaner' direction, not dissimilar to trends identified in the private manufacturing sector (Womack et al, 1990). Nevertheless, it is clear from these accounts that some degree of professional autonomy is preserved, both in the choice of knowledge being employed and in the discretion used in its operationalisation in particular cases. This is not the programmed and routinised reduction of complex problems to simplistic solutions. The negotiated, relational and collaborative application of the professionals' knowledge and judgment is emphasised.

What comes across from the protagonists of the approach is a missionary zeal. There is only a rare glimpse of ambivalence, as in the comment of one consultant social worker (Goodman and Trowler, 2012, p 88) that 'systemic social work is exhausting. It requires a sensitive and humorous unit or team to make up for the stress of the individual worker.... It is crucial that the whole unit continuously discusses and reviews the course of action and that the individual worker has the same goal as the rest of the unit.' However, according to the same source, the system frees up far more time for emotional support for staff than the traditional model (Goodman and Trowler, 2012, p 88). Reflection on cases takes place in the unit meetings while supervision sessions can focus far more on individual staff development. 'In our model of work, supervision is a core factor for successful retainment [sic] of emotional resources' (Goodman and Trowler, 2012, p 88). Moreover, from the point of view of one of the participants in a 'children practitioner's role' (Goodman and Trowler, 2012, p 135), the model involves: 'The reclaiming of a sense of direction, of confidence, of expertise and of gravitas in the way we go about our work.' These are big claims, and, if justified, suggest a 'reclaiming' that brings greater professional autonomy to social work, both in the way the profession organises itself and in the everyday practice and experience of the individual social worker.

There is little doubt that implementing this model did bring about significant change in the organisation in which it was first developed – Hackney's children's services. This was a change management process led from the top, by transformative, if not charismatic, leaders. They worked out a model that seemed to be embraced by those who operated it with some degree of enthusiasm. It should be noted, however, that, even in the account of the leaders there is reference to people leaving, with even some of those recruited to implement the changes having 'fallen by the wayside, disappointed by their misinterpretation or our mis-represenation of how things would be' (Goodman and Trowler, 2012, p 168).

The book on which this review of the Hackney model is based is hardly a disinterested account. It presents a story of success and may be a one-sided representation, even if it is a collaborative effort, with chapters written by people with different roles in the organisation. If it receives support from researchers such as in the Munro report (2011), this, too, might be interpreted as coming from within a subset of the professional group who are 'believers' – in this case believers in relationship-based social work. The book is based on a clear narrative – the failure of the recent, heavily bureaucratic model. What the alternative does, though, is not eliminate evidence-based practice or managerialism, but seek to organise it in such a way as to enhance relationship-based social work. It can be seen as a (re-)professionalising project that is certainly challenging the kind of 'proletarianising' trends identified by Carey but might not be a fundamental challenge to a neoliberal mindset that seeks efficiency and 'lean' public agencies above all else. Indeed the model could ultimately lend itself to the outsourcing of social work in voluntary or private organisations applying such principles. Such an outcome would be anathema to another author who used the 'reclaiming social work' phrase – Iain Ferguson (2008) - and it is to his work that we turn next.

Alternative 3: reclaiming social work – type 2

Ferguson (2008) articulates a radical alternative to what he sees as 'neoliberal' social work practice. His analysis of the situation in which social workers are cast is similar to that of the other analyses presented here – the managerialisation of social work is seen as stifling social work's potential to do good, making the job of the social worker more constrained and less satisfying. Ferguson points to signs of dissatisfaction with – and resistance to – neoliberal social work. This comes in a number of tangible forms such as critical conferences, marches, meetings and manifestos.

Ferguson's is not a parochial UK-centred view; rather he sees the inspiration for a reconfiguration of social work in a radical direction as prompted as much from developments from outside the UK – particularly from Australia, Canada and South America – as from within the UK. For Ferguson, the radical alternative to contemporary social work rests on the values of respect, empowerment and social justice (Ferguson, 2008). Ferguson argues that social work needs to reach out and support other social movements such as the mental health service user movement. To Ferguson, the alternative to neoliberal social work is radical and political. As he notes, this is not particularly new, having some continuity with attempts to radicalise social work in the UK in the 1920s, as well as with the radical social work ideas promoted in the 1970s.

The changes he advocates are presented as a kind of 'socialism from below'. It is based on user involvement, not as 'consumers' but as citizens engaged in collective attempts to bring about change and social justice. Ferguson is critical of what he describes as 'narrow' interpretations of 'critical' social work, something he associates with postmodernism, which he sees as leading to a more individualised and particular set of practices, ignoring 'structural' features. He prefers a broader interpretation, which has as its emphasis collective action rooted in structural factors. If it is a relationship-based model, this is not the relationships of psychodynamics and family therapies, but of networking and organising for change. In this model the social worker is cast as facilitator and activist – if there is a degree of autonomy, it would seem to come from being able to decide on who, when and how to support, represent and mobilise others – these are political rather than 'evidence-based' or 'evidence-informed' knowledges of a psycho-technicist nature. This, too, might be seen as a relational autonomy; one based on partnerships and networked governance.

Conclusion

This chapter has presented three different routes away from a managerial-technicist version of social work. While rooted in UK debates and practice it might be used by social workers in other countries as pointing to different alternatives, three different ways of doing things: the first, reconfiguring professional practice in the direction of evaluation in practice; the second 'reclaiming social work' on the Hackney relationship-based model; and the third 'reclaiming social work' in a more radical, highly politicised way. The first set of ideas is influential in the academy and not without appeal to social workers who might feel beleaguered, belittled and denigrated. It offers some dignity and occupational control. However, it confronts at least two difficulties: first, the relentless pace of work that makes reflection and evaluation in practice more difficult, and, second, the difficulty of articulating and agreeing a moral purpose. Perhaps social workers today would generally subscribe to an ethics of care, of positive relationships based on trust, respect, openness and dialogue, and this might distinguish contemporary social workers from their 19th-century forerunners, rooted in the pursuit of discipline, sobriety and industry. But such moral values are perhaps more easily seen as the basis for relationships with colleagues, service users, and other care professionals than for bringing about substantial social change.

If autonomy has been a theme running through this chapter, the questions it raises are not just those of how much autonomy social workers have in different models, but also of what kind and for what purpose. All three might be said to rest on 'relational' forms of autonomy, rather than a more traditional model of professional dominance, but each suggests a different interpretation of relational autonomy and of the moral purpose of social work. If the moral purpose remains undefined in the first alternative, perhaps, in the Hackney model the moral purpose has been reduced to a minimum: the need to safeguard the child. This model could represent something of a compromise that achieves efficiency and effectiveness with some degree of professional autonomy. However, this would seem to be a relatively modest achievement – a 'reclaiming' for social work of a 'relationship-based' form that has at its root a limited set of ambitions – the safeguarding of children from the worst forms of abuse and neglect.

Ferguson's vision of a more radical social work would seem to be more at odds with the dominant ideology of the time. For this reason, it is difficult to see the state providing the funds for such a radical form of activism. If there is hope for this, it perhaps rests in civil society rather than within the state – in voluntary associations and networks of activists rather than the ranks of salaried 'social workers'. But then history has a way of springing surprises on us.

References

Aberdeen City Council (2014) 'Aberdeen children's services set for major boost', available at www.aberdeencity.gov.uk/CouncilNews/ci_cns/pr_reclaimsocialwork_110913.asp (accessed 22 June 2016).

Ackroyd, S. and Thompson, P. (1999) *Organizational misbehaviour*, London: Sage Publications.

Aronson, J. and Smith, K. (2011) 'Identity work and critical social service management: balancing on a tightrope?', *British Journal of Social Work*, 41: 432-48.

Carey, M. (2009) '"It's like being a robot or working in a factory": does Braverman help explain the experience of state social workers in Britain since 1971?', *Organization*, 16(4): 505-27.

Clarke, J. (2004) 'Dissolving the public realm? The logics and limits of neo-liberalism', *Journal of Social Policy*, 33(1): 27-48.

Clarke, J. and Newman, J. (1997) *The managerial state*, London: Sage Publications.

Community Care (2013) 'Troubled council scraps reclaiming social work model', available at www.communitycare.co.uk/2013/09/26/troubled-council-scraps-reclaiming-social-work-model/#.UymK9IV-nuo (accessed 22 June 2016).

Evans, T. (2011) 'Professionals, managers and discretion: critiquing street-level bureaucracy', *British Journal of Social Work*, 41(2): 368-86.

Evans, T. and Harris, J. (2004) 'Street-level bureaucracy, social work and the (exaggerated) death of discretion', *British Journal of Social Work*, 34(6): 871-95.

Ferguson, I. (2008) *Reclaiming social work: Challenging neo-liberalism and promoting social justice*, London: Sage Publications.

Goodman, S. and Trowler, I. (2012) *Social work reclaimed: Innovative frameworks for child and family social work*, London: Jessica Kingsley.

Gupta, A. and Blewett, J. (2007) 'Change for children? The challenges and opportunities for the children's social work workforce', *Child & Family Social Work*, 12(2): 172-81.

Harlow, E. (2003) 'New managerialism, social services departments and social work practice today', *Practice*, 15(2): 29-44.

Harlow, E. (2004) 'Why don't women want to be social workers anymore? New managerialism, postfeminism and the shortage of social workers in social services departments in England and Wales', *European Journal of Social Work*, 7(2): 167-80.
Harlow, E., Berg, E., Barry, J. and Chandler, J. (2013) 'Neoliberalism, managerialism and the reconfiguring of social work in Sweden and the United Kingdom', *Organization*, 20(4): 534-50.
Hood, C. (1991) 'Public management for all seasons?', *Public Administration*, 69(1): 3-19.
Lymbery, M. (2001) 'Social work at the crossroads', *British Journal of Social Work*, 31(3): 369-84.
Mackenzie, C. and Stoljar, N. (eds) (2000) *Relational autonomy: Feminist perspectives on automony, agency, and the social self*, Oxford: Oxford University Press.
Munro, E. (2011) *The Munro review of child protection: Final report*, Norwich: The Stationery Office.
Peters, T. and Waterman, R.H. (1982) *In search of excellence: Lessons from America's best run companies*, New York, NY: Harper and Row.
Pollitt, C. (1990) *Managerialism and the public services: The Anglo-American experience*, Oxford: Blackwell.
Power, M.P. (1997) *The audit society: Rituals of verification*, Oxford: Oxford University Press.
Schedler, K. and Proeller, I. (2002) 'The new public management: A perspective from mainland Europe', in K. McLaughlin, S.P. Osborne and E. Ferlie (eds) *New Public Management: Current trends and future prospects*, London: Routledge.
Shaw, I. (2011) *Evaluating in practice*, Farnham: Ashgate.
White, S. (2009) *Error, blame and responsibility in child welfare: Problematics of governance in an invisible trade: Full Research Report*, ESRC End of Award Report, RES-166-25-0048-A, Swindon: Economic and Social Research Council.
Womack, J.P. Jones, D.T. and Roos, J. (1990) *The machine that changed the world*, Oxford: Maxwell Macmillan International.

SIX

Auditing and accountability

Anders Hanberger, Lena Lindgren and Lennart Nygren

This chapter consists of two parts. First, two accountability dilemmas are identified, key concepts are defined, and a framework for exploring the interplay among democratic governance, audit systems and accountability is presented. Second, two different but dominant audit systems used in Swedish eldercare are described and analysed in light of this framework, and consequences of auditing and accountability for key actors involved are discussed, as well as possible ways of resolving the two accountability dilemmas. In relation to the volume, this chapter explores conditions, trends and challenges in today's audit society and their implications for welfare professions and other key actors. Swedish eldercare is an illustrative case of a phenomenon occurring in most policy sectors.

Introduction

According to the political theorist John Keane (2008), there has been a fundamental shift in representative democracy since the Second World War towards a form of 'monitory democracy' defined by the multiplication and dispersal of multiple power-monitoring and power-contesting mechanisms, within both the domestic and cross-border fields of government and civil society. Various forms of audit exemplify such mechanisms. Audit as an organisational and democratic control function was first confined to the financial examination of accounts. However, an audit explosion in recent decades has extended the concept and the ways governments and organisations undertake various kinds of audits, such as supervision, financial and performance audits (Power, 1997; Dahler-Larsen, 2012).

The 1990s saw growing demands for governments to achieve better results in public policies, agencies and services, and performance assessment is now an indispensable component of various New Public Management (NPM) regimes (Radin, 2006; Van Dooren et al, 2010). NPM needs recurrent performance information about the quality of actions and about what these actions have achieved in order to fine tune and control implementation, monitor and assess the achievement of objectives, hold lower levels to account, and create a sense of control (Behn, 2001). To meet these needs, numerous new audit systems have been established and prevailing ones have received new attention in many sectors of the welfare state worldwide, not least in human services organisations (Munro, 2004; Clarkson and Challis, 2006; Johansson et al, 2015).

Two dilemmas

Although NPM reforms have created new ways of visualising desirable results that emphasise the role of audits in supporting accountability for performance, this is not the only form of accountability found in democratic governance. Governments and their agencies are still accountable for finances and fairness. This creates an accountability dilemma for public managers in that they cannot simultaneously improve performance, follow the rules and regulations, and stay within their budgets (Behn, 2001). To avoid being criticised in audits, most managers will before anything else ensure that they are 'audit-proof', that is, that they are complying with rules and keeping within their budgets. If time, resources, and capacity allow, they will make efforts to enhance performance.

Policymakers generally expect a great deal from auditing, at least according to their rhetoric, while professionals tend to expect less or even resist auditing. We argue that this reflects a tension between auditing for political (that is, hierarchical) accountability, which implies that the performance of social services is being monitored against politically and administratively predefined standards (Behn, 2001), and professional accountability, in which good performance is based on trust that the professional agent is qualified to make situated judgments and improve practice (Evetts, 2009; Evans, 2011). While auditing for political accountability conveys an inbuilt distrust of professionals, it nevertheless relies on professionals to improve the performance of services (Van Dooren et al, 2010). The second dilemma thus implies balancing the monitoring of performance against the risk of generating professional distrust.

Purpose

Along with the development of NPM, a wealth of literature focuses on governance, audit and accountability. The purpose here is to use this literature to compile a conceptual framework for exploring the interplay among governance, audit systems and accountability in today's audit societies and human service organisations. The framework is then employed in analysing the two most important national audit systems in Swedish eldercare – state supervision and Open Comparisons – which are used as illustrative examples to highlight general critical aspects and consequences for key actors of auditing for accountability in human service organisations. The chapter ends with conclusions about consequences of the audit systems for the key actors and about how the two dilemmas might be resolved.

Conceptual framework and methods

The *audit society* refers to a set of attitudes or cultural commitments to problem solving in which evaluation, checking and accountability are expected conduct in collective action (Power, 1997). *Auditing* can take on various forms. State supervision, financial and performance audit, evaluation, accreditation and performance measurement are all evaluative activities concerned in different ways with assessing the performance of governmental programmes and agencies (Johansson and Lindgren, 2013; OECD/EU, 2013). *Audit system* refers to the procedural, institutional and policy arrangements shaping the audit function and its relationship to its internal and external environment (Liverani and Lundgren, 2007, p 241).

The meaning of *accountability* has been extended in several directions (Mulgan, 2000; Behn, 2001; Bovens, 2010). The traditional notion of accountability as external scrutiny and counting is based on the assumption of a clear distinction between politics and administration (Finer, 1941). According to Behn (2001), democratic accountability includes accountability for finances, fairness and performance.

Accountability for finances implies that those in power can explain what they have done with taxpayers' money and will not exceed budgets, and are held accountable for following the rules and spending the money as intended. *Accountability for fairness* suggests that those in power or the relevant responsible organisations have paid due attention to ethical standards such as fairness and equity. Rules and procedural standards are set for the values organisations are to pay attention to, and to create expectations. There is also a need to hold government and public organisations accountable for the discharge, outcome and consequences of public policy – in other words, *accountability for performance*. There must be expectations according to which performance can be assessed, and setting such expectations is a critical matter in a democracy. For whom and against which standard should governmental or organisational performance be assessed? There is no consensus about which performance criteria to use in assessing public policies. From a democratic governance perspective, three possible solutions to the criteria dilemma can be identified: criteria can be selected and justified as supporting national government, local government, or key actors.

Table 6.1: Framework for exploring auditing and accountability in eldercare governance

Governance model	*Audit system*	*Kinds of accountability*	*Consequences for key actors*
State Local government Multi-actor	State supervision Performance measurement	Finances Fairness Performance	Decision makers Care providers Professionals Users

Sources: Behn (2001); Hanberger (2009, 2011)

Against this background, the conceptual framework depicted in Table 6.1 has been compiled to guide the description of audit systems and support the analysis of critical aspects and consequences for key actors. The framework conceives of auditing (in this chapter, state supervision and performance measurement) from a governance perspective, that is, as support for state, local government, or multi-actor governance. As this chapter is focused on auditing and accountability, the role of auditing in democratic governance is paid extra attention. Three kinds of accountability – for finances, fairness and performance – are examined. From having an accountability function, auditing can promote further democratic functions, such as eldercare policy, improvement and legitimisation (Behn, 2001; Van Dooren et al, 2008). Audit systems used for political accountability can have different consequences for the key actors; for example, decision makers can be forced to take action they do not believe is right if service organisations do not meet expectations, whereas professionals may need to prioritise what is being measured even if it does not correspond to professional ethics and guidelines.

Three data sources constitute the empirical basis of this chapter, namely, policy documents, texts from the websites of the Health and Social Care Inspectorate (IVO), the National Board of Health and

Welfare (NBHW), and the Swedish Association of Local Authorities and Regions (SALAR), and interviews with staff involved in running the state supervision (SSV) of eldercare and Open Comparisons (OC).

The character and function of two audit systems in Swedish eldercare

State supervision

IVO is a central government agency responsible for supervising healthcare and social services, including eldercare, since June 2013. IVO is also responsible for issuing certain permits in these areas. Its supervision responsibility covers the processing of complaints concerning, for example, the reporting of irregularities in healthcare and social care and the municipal obligation to report non-enforced decisions (www.ivo.se). The dividing lines between the responsibilities of various providers are sometimes unclear. This means that IVO does not just examine individual services, but also considers how the whole care chain functions and whether and how collaboration takes place between providers. Eldercare supervision covers special eldercare homes and homecare services for the elderly. IVO operates as a compliance-monitoring actor within the *state model of governance* (Table 6.1).

The audit system for eldercare supervision has been developed as part of IVO's general commission. The audit system consists of desktop supervision as well as preannounced and unannounced inspections. IVO's general commission, special government assignments for issue-focused supervision, and laws and regulations for eldercare guide SSV. Eldercare supervision, which applies a user perspective, monitors compliance with the Health and Medical Services Act and other national eldercare standards. IVO states that supervision requires independent and free-standing examination to confirm that laws and other regulations are being followed.

The core of eldercare SSV is accountability for fairness and accountability for performance. All citizens are to receive good eldercare on equal terms irrespective of where in the country they live. Individual care receivers or their relatives must be able to be sure that the Act is being followed and that their interests are being safeguarded. It is important to be able to count on compliance with the rules concerning processing, safety, equal treatment, and the right to particular services.

For each supervision, a decision is issued specifying insufficiencies and any needed improvement actions. A yearly summary report is compiled for all supervisions with conclusions regarding the state of eldercare and needs for action. IVO uses both soft methods (dialogue, interviews, and good examples) and hard methods (fines and facility closure) in its supervision. As a result, SSV supervisees are expected to take action before and after inspection to comply with laws and regulations and to resolve identified problems. SSV is assumed to ensure a minimum level of eldercare service according to national standards and to ensure that the elderly are provided safe, high-quality eldercare and services.

Although instrumental compliance with the statutes can be expected shortly before preannounced supervisions or after supervisions that identify poor conditions and violations of statutes, the effects of these supervisions will probably not be long-lasting or have much effect on uninspected care providers (SSV is performed only on selected care providers).

Open Comparisons

Since 2007, NBHW has collaborated with SALAR in publishing annual performance information known as Open Comparisons (OC) in numerous social service areas, including eldercare, the focus of this chapter. The overall aim of OC is to improve the performance of social services by increasing transparency and providing open access to comparable information on quality, results and costs. Subordinate objectives are to provide better opportunities for management and control and to support well-informed choices of social care provider. The primary targeted users of the information are public managers and politicians in local authorities, while service users and citizens, stakeholder organisations and the news media are secondary target groups.

Around 35 indicators are used to assess the performance of eldercare services at the municipal level, and some of these indicators apply at the unit level as well. In annual reports, municipalities are compared and ranked using a relative green, yellow and red scale. The indicators are based on data from four data sources: official statistics, recurrent user satisfaction surveys, and patient and pharmacy registers. The indicators constitute measures of eldercare service performance based on NBHW's and SALAR's interpretation and operationalisation of eldercare requirements and objectives specified in laws and other provisions, and of resources assumed to be needed to accomplish them. Of the 35 indicators, more than half measure activities and outputs; most of the rest measure the resources that care providers have at their disposal and a few measure the effects of care on the lives of service users.

Regarding the conceptual framework employed in this chapter, OC represents a performance measurement type of audit system, intended mainly to provide governance support in the areas of activity for which local governments (municipalities and county councils) are accountable. However, OC has been developed and is administered by a central government agency (NBHW) in collaboration with SALAR, which is formally a non-governmental organisation that represents and advocates the interests of local governments. In terms of governance model, OC eldercare exemplifies multi-actor governance in which a semi-governmental organisation and a state agency collaborate in developing and running the audit system.

The kind of accountability sought through OC is mainly accountability for performance – that is, the quality of activities and outputs – and to a lesser extent for what has been achieved because of these activities and outputs – effects. Some of the indicators measuring resources (such as staff continuity and service accessibility) could in practice be connected with accountability for fairness.

In the next section, the consequences of the two audit systems presented here are discussed for each of the four key actors in the conceptual framework, with a focus on what are considered critical aspects of auditing for accountability. We then return to the two dilemmas described in the introduction – namely, that managers cannot simultaneously improve performance, follow the rules and regulations, and stay within their budgets, and that accountability for performance presupposes professionals' involvement and commitment, but also implies lack of trust in them – and explore how they can be managed and possibly resolved.

Consequences for key actors

Decision makers

Sweden is a welfare state with several responsibilities decentralised to the local level. Local self-government is strongly protected (Montin, 2007) and gives municipalities substantial discretion to adapt eldercare to local conditions and needs. National decision makers (that is, politicians and officials) and local decision makers in the municipalities have different roles in eldercare governance. National decision makers operate within the current statutes for eldercare, but they can also take action to change laws and regulations if they think there is a need. The institutionalisation of IVO in 2013 is an example of such a change. Local decision makers are responsible for implementing national eldercare policy and must comply with the statutes, but they can use their discretion to choose a feasible organisational form for eldercare and to allow or disallow private service providers.

The two audit systems provide the decision makers at both levels with complementary performance information for results-based eldercare governance. OC produces input and performance data and SSV produces compliance data.

The consequence of OC for national decision makers is that they must respond to how the 35 performance indicators play out in public and private eldercare around the country, in both small and large municipalities. They also need to respond to IVO's summary reports on SSV of eldercare in the country at large, and take action if problems are identified. They can use information from both systems to hold agencies and municipalities to account for compliance with the statutes and for achieving national objectives for eldercare, and take action to improve eldercare if needed.

The attention decision makers have to pay to the performance information depends on the results: negative results generally demand more action than do positive results. How the media present the results is also of importance, as are the expectations for political action and the way in which decision makers in power prioritise eldercare issues.

Local decision makers also have to respond to the same indicators, in particular to the results reflecting inter-municipality differences and how other similar municipalities perform when benchmarked. The public reporting of OC, combined with the green-yellow-red ranking of municipalities with reference to the 35 performance indicators, holds local politicians accountable, prompting them to act in response to the indicators to avoid being red-flagged in the future. Holding actors accountable in this way, or rather making them feel accountable, is based on a naming-and-shaming mechanism that is considered very powerful (Pawson, 2002).

If a municipal eldercare supervision reveals problems relating to quality, politicians in power are held accountable for these insufficiencies and must respond to IVO's critique. This response includes reacting to and managing sanctions. SSV and OC entail strengthening municipalities as agents of the state, although they are accountable to their local citizens.

A *critical aspect* of OC is that the performance measures are only partly valid and not always reliable, especially not at a disaggregated level. Decision makers have to rely on summary reports and assume that SALAR and OC have measured and compared the problems so that aggregated performance measures reflect real differences in eldercare provision and quality. If performance measures are invalid or only partly valid, decision makers will base their decisions and action on misconceptions of eldercare conditions.

A critical aspect of state supervision is that SSV reports focus on eldercare compliance with the statutes, but provide little information on eldercare that actually works well. SSV provides decision makers with reports on multiple supervisions, and on eldercare at risk of not complying with the statutes. The share of eldercare homes and homecare service providers that is supervised is small, and is based on a selection of care providers and municipalities (based on risk assessment) that may not reflect eldercare as a whole.

If decision makers overemphasise the use of OC performance measures for benchmarking, they could become victims of the audit system themselves, that is, they must continually consider what to do with municipalities that perform below average. The red, yellow, and green signals hinder them from monitoring progress.

To resolve the first dilemma (that managers cannot simultaneously improve performance, follow the rules and regulations, and stay within their budgets), local politicians must create a feasible and effective organisation, adhere to the budget, and comply with the statutes. They also need to provide fair conditions for professionals, and listen to and support both the professionals and eldercare providers. If not, there will be no latitude to improve eldercare performance.

The second dilemma (that accountability for performance presupposes professionals' involvement and commitment, but implies lack of trust in them) may be resolved if local politicians avoid using OC and SSV instrumentally, consider more information and knowledge than just the supervision results, and let the professionals work professionally.

Care providers

Before the 1990s, eldercare in Sweden was regarded as an entirely public (municipal) matter, but many municipalities have since outsourced parts of their eldercare services to private providers or introduced a consumer-choice system. This has created a market-like situation in which elderly people choose services from various public and private care providers. For this key actor, significant consequences are linked to reputation and rewards. If care providers are rated poorly in OC eldercare or in IVO inspection reports, their reputations are impaired. On the other hand, if their performance is rated above average, they can use this fact for promotion.

A critical aspect for care providers is that it is generally difficult to transform actual eldercare into predefined categories, including the OC performance indicators. The most important aspects of eldercare are not measurable or difficult to measure. As incentives and resources are linked to performance measures, there is a risk of unintended effects, such as threshold effects, ratchet effects and output distortion (Hood, 2012). Care providers have to deliver input, output and performance data not only to OC but also to Statistics Sweden, the municipal eldercare department, and also the owner of eldercare companies. The required documentation and reporting takes time from actual eldercare work.

Another critical aspect concerns the diverse conditions under which public and private providers work. In relation to IVO, public providers are required to report serious deficiencies through the local government's committee responsible for eldercare, while private providers do the reporting by themselves. In addition, the right of staff to act as whistleblowers is stronger in public organisations (where the employer is prohibited from seeking out the person who revealed the information) than in private organisations (Erlandsson et al, 2013).

The first dilemma (that managers cannot simultaneously improve performance, follow the rules and regulations, and stay within their budgets) can be resolved to some extent, but not fully, if care providers are properly organised and budgets are adhered to, in which case there may be room for improvement. Providers that have already developed high-quality care, however, cannot improve much more but must strive to maintain quality. The second dilemma, concerning the need for professionals' commitment but lack of trust in them, can be expected to play out differently between public and private care providers, because it appears that sanctions are stronger for staff in private organisations. Consequently, private care providers and staff may hesitate to blow the whistle even if there are severe problems in the workplace or organisation.

Professionals

A core characteristic of professional work is that the profession is entrusted with responsibility for defining the standards of what constitutes good work – that is, professional accountability – here, in eldercare (Evans, 2011). This trust relies on the premise that professionals, through academic training and vocational experience, are qualified to handle problems responsibly, deliver good service efficiently, and apply discretionary reasoning in practice. However, some kind of external control of professionals is still needed, though the functioning of SSV, performance measurement systems (OC) and other strategies employed by NPM tends to overlook professional knowledge and accountability in favor of politically predefined and universal standards of good eldercare work – that is, political accountability (Evetts, 2009).

Although the distinction between professional and political accountability is not as sharp in practice as it may seem to be in theory, the trend towards political accountability has consequences for the development of professional practice. Being held accountable against politically predefined and universal standards assumes that eldercare professionals can improve their performance by adhering to these standards, that is, through single-loop learning. However, rigid accountability systems and single-loop learning and improvement strategies tend to drive out double-loop learning (Argyris and Schön, 1996) in which improvement is not simply a matter of conformity but of having the capacity to respond appropriately – and professionally – by making the changes required. In the long run, this single-loop dynamic will lower the professional status of eldercare work, possibly deprofessionalising eldercare workers who are pressured to act in standardised ways while devaluing the essential elements of professional practice (Randall et al, 1999).

The dilemma that managers cannot simultaneously improve performance, follow rules and regulations, and stay within their budgets can be resolved if managers succeed in applying the approach discussed here. The second dilemma, that accountability for performance presupposes professionals' involvement and commitment but implies a lack of trust in the professionals, is trickier to resolve. Given the discrepancy between single- and double-loop learning, implementing accountability for performance through measurement and state supervision is probably not the best way to improve performance. A management strategy for double-loop learning and performance improvement would entail giving professionals the latitude to question established routines and seek innovative solutions. However, with such a strategy, there is also a need to devise other information sources to supplement, or substitute for, performance measurement data.

Users

Users are expected to participate in improving the quality of care services in Sweden (Kjellberg, 2012). This is reflected only partly in the two systems discussed in this chapter. Users who are dissatisfied or maltreated can make direct use of SSV through formal complaint procedures. Serious medical maltreatment must be reported to IVO by the care provider according to a specific law, lex Maria. The corresponding law for social care, lex Sarah, makes it obligatory to report deficiencies (or risks of serious deficiencies) and for the care provider to take action. Serious lex Maria cases must be reported to IVO (Erlandsson et al, 2013). Actions taken by care providers due to complaints imply direct consequences for the user.

Regarding OC, the relevance to users is indirect. OC contains user satisfaction indicators (e.g. treatment, service, and security). In the best case, one possible consequence is that the care provider adapts to negative OC results by allocating more resources to the problem area. Another consequence is that OC information can guide users when choosing care providers. In addition, users can mobilise the media based on OC results, and can combine OC information with personal witness testimony to put pressure on local decision-makers and eldercare providers.

For IVO, a *critical aspect* is whether users have enough information about how to make complaints and about the actions they can expect from the care providers. The process for addressing complaints after receiving them is underdeveloped in many municipalities, and only a minority of municipalities has developed procedures for managing feedback to the user (Harnett, 2010). This deficiency means that the responsibility for following up on complaints has passed to the users and their families.

Regarding OC, a critical aspect is that even if the system provides information, the choice of care provider can be an empty choice as there are too few alternative choices in small municipalities: few nursing homes have been built so users end up waiting for care in provisional homes or in their own homes.

Users are not directly part of the dilemma of having to perform well and follow rules and regulations while adhering to budgets. Just as users can become 'hostages' in the struggle between political and professional accountability, they can also become 'weapons' in budget fights between decision makers and professionals when limited resources threaten desirable performance (the second dilemma). One final question recalls the professional commitment/mistrust dilemma: How much will decision makers – and professionals – trust the involvement of users in care planning and quality improvement?

Conclusion

Both audit systems share certain important consequences for key eldercare actors (as in the case reported here), but there are also identifiable differences. All actors have to respond to performance measures (OC) that are not completely valid and trustworthy, and all need to consider interventions that work well in eldercare together with reports of bad conditions identified in SSV to avoid being captured and governed by numbers and targets alone. They also have to manage unintended effects such as output distortion manifested as targetisation (Hood, 2012).

Professionals are subjected to external and internal accountability pressure, to which they must learn to respond and for which they must develop response strategies while balancing this against professional accountability. Governments and citizens cannot hand over all control to the professions because this does not guarantee that public resources will not be misused. The state monitors and controls professionals on behalf of citizens because they too are stakeholders. Although professionals claim to be doing what is best for their clients, according to what they have learned as professionals (Abbott, 1988), this tends to coincide with their own interests. Accordingly, both public and private eldercare need to be subjected to national scrutiny and recurrent monitoring and control.

The two dilemmas could possibly be resolved if decision makers and service providers developed feasible and effective organisations and used the two audit systems critically in combination with other knowledge and information, including their own common sense. They must also try to balance their political accountability obligations and regulatory audit regimes against the principles and codes of professional accountability obligations in order to prevent or at least reduce negative effects such as targetisation and deprofessionalisation. A balance must be struck between professional discretion and democratic control. Granting more freedom to professionals, unaccompanied by democratic control, could ultimately lead to meritocracy. The challenge is to develop well-adjusted political accountability that avoids deprofessionalisation without relinquishing democratic control.

References

Abbott, A. (1988) *The system of professions. An essay on the division of expert labor*, Chicago, IL: University of Chicago Press.

Argyris, C. and Schön, D. (1996) *Organizational learning II: Theory, method and practice*, Reading, MA: Addison-Wesley.

Behn, R. (2001) *Rethinking democratic accountability*, Washington, D.C.: Brookings Institution Press.

Bovens, M. (2010) 'Two concepts of accountability: accountability as a virtue and as a mechanism', *West European Politics*, 33(5): 946-67.

Clarkson, P. and Challis, D. (2006) 'Performance measurement in social care: a comparison of efficiency measurement methods', *Social Policy and Society*, 5(4): 461-77.

Dahler-Larsen, P. (2012) *The evaluation society*, Stanford, CA: Stanford Business Books.

Erlandsson, S., Storm, P., Stranz, A., Szebehely, M. and Trydegård, G. (2013) 'Marketising trends in Swedish eldercare: competition, choice and calls for stricter regulation', in G. Meagher and M. Szehebely (eds) *Marketisation in Nordic eldercare. A research report on legislation, oversight, extent and consequences*, Stockholm: Stockholm University, Department of Social Work, pp 23-83.

Evans, T. (2011) 'Professionals, managers and discretion: critiquing street-level bureaucracy', *British Journal of Social Work*, 41(2): 368-86.

Evetts, J. (2009) 'New professionalism and New Public Management: changes, continuities and consequences', *Comparative Sociology*, 8(2): 247-66.

Finer, H. (1941) 'Administrative responsibility in democratic government', *Public Administration Review*, 1(4): 335-50.

Hanberger, A. (2009) 'Democratic accountability in decentralized governance', *Scandinavian Political Studies*, 32(1): 1-22.

Hanberger, A. (2011) 'The real functions of evaluation and response systems', *Evaluation*, 17(4): 327-49.

Harnett, T. (2010) *The trivial matters. Everyday power in Swedish elder care*, Jönköping: Jönköping University.

Hood, C. (2012) 'Public management by numbers as a performance-enhancing drug: two hypotheses', *Public Administration Review*, 72(1): 85-92.

Johansson, S., Dellgran, P. and Höjer, S. (eds) (2015) *Människobehandlande organisationer. Villkor för ledning, styrning och professionellt välfärdsarbete* [Human services organizations. Conditions for the leadership, management and professional welfare work], Stockholm: Natur & Kultur.

Johansson, V. and Lindgren, L. (2013) *Uppdrag offentlig granskning* [Assignment – public scrutiny], Lund: Studentlitteratur.

Keane, J. (2008) 'Monitory democracy', Paper presented at the ESRC Seminar Series, Emergent Publics, The Open University, Milton Keynes, 13-14 March.

Kjellberg, I. (2012) *Klagomålshantering och lex Sarah-rapportering i äldreomsorgen. En institutionell etnografisk studie* [Complaints and lex Sarah-reporting in elderly care. An institutional ethnographic study], Gothenburg: Gothenburg University, Department of Social Work.

Liverani, A. and Lundgren, H. (2007) 'Evaluation systems in development aid agencies. An analysis of DAC peer reviews 1996-2004', *Evaluation*, 13(2): 241-56.

Montin, S. (2007) *Moderna kommuner* [Modern municipalities] (3rd edn), Malmö: Liber.

Mulgan, R. (2000) 'Accountability: an ever-expanding concept?', *Public Administration*, 78(3): 555-73.

Munro, E. (2004) 'The impact of audit on social work practice', *British Journal of Social Work*, 34(8): 1075-95.

OECD/EU (Organisation for Economic Co-operation and Development/European Union) (2013) *A good life in old age? Monitoring and improving quality in long-term care*, OECD Health Policy Studies, Paris: OECD.

Pawson, R. (2002) 'Evidence and policy and naming and shaming', *Policy Studies*, 23(3-4): 211-30.

Power, M. (1997) *The audit society: Rituals of verification*, Oxford: Oxford University Press.

Radin, B.A. (2006) *Challenging the performance movement. Accountability, complexity and democratic values*, Washington, DC: Georgetown University Press.

Randall, M.L., Cropanzano, R., Bormann, C.A. and Birjulin, A. (1999) 'Organizational politics and organizational support as predictors of work attitudes, job performance, and organizational citizenship behavior', *Journal of Organizational Behavior*, 20: 159-74.

Van Dooren, W. and Van de Walle, S. (eds) (2008) *Performance information in the public sector. How it is used*, Basingstoke: Palgrave MacMillan.

Van Dooren, W., Bouckaert, G. and Halligan, J. (2010) *Performance management in the public sector*, Abingdon: Routledge.

SEVEN

State regulation of the social work profession: an example from Poland

Kazimiera Wódz and Krystyna Faliszek

Introduction

The aim of this chapter is to discuss how the development and professionalisation of social work can be regulated by the state through jurisdiction and standardisation. We do this by focusing on the situation in Poland after the political transformation that started in 1989, assuming such demarcation seems justified if we observe the exceptionally unfavourable circumstances for social work existing in Poland in the years 1945-89. In describing the most important factors that influenced the formation of social work as an academic discipline and a field of practice from the beginning of the 1990s, we do not neglect or diminish the existing traditions and achievements of the earlier generations of pedagogues, charity organisation activists and academics who from the late 1920s were engaged in the development of social work in Poland. However, development in Poland since 1990 has undoubtedly brought an unprecedented growth in the number of universities offering curricula in social work – not like before as a specialisation within pedagogical sciences (social pedagogy) or sociology, but as a separate programme. The introduction of diplomas in social work (Bachelor of Social Work, and Master's programmes) was a milestone in turning social work into a 'mature profession',[1] but it was not the only factor shaping the public image and professional practice of the growing number of qualified social workers. The second, even more important, factor was legislation, especially in the field of social welfare; first of all the Social Assistance Act (1990) and a number of laws and administrative regulations of social security introduced in subsequent years. The main thesis in this chapter is that the development of professional social work was influenced mainly by the state (government) policies, with limited support from the representatives of social work partners (non-governmental organisations, or NGOs), practitioners and academics. The 'modernisation' of social services delivery was undertaken in the years 2007-13, within the Operational Programme of Human Capital Development (POKL). This effort, co-financed by the European Social Fund, was focused mainly on the 'standardisation' of social work as a way to raise the efficiency of social services in fighting social exclusion. As we show, there was a counter-effect to standardisation, which tends to lead to diminished autonomy of professional social workers' community. We argue that this strive for standardisation of social work practice, initiated by central government (Ministry of Labour and Social Policy), is partly inspired by New Public Management, pro-market, neoliberal ideologies, with the hidden aim to limit the direct involvement of the public sector in social services delivery.

Theoretical assumptions

The professional status of social work has been a matter of many debates since the early 20th century. There is not enough space here for a comprehensive overview of the literature on this issue (see Flexner, 1915; Greenwood, 1957; Wenocur and Reisch, 1983; Abbott, 1988, 1995). However, we would like to mention two main approaches developed by scholars studying the professionalism of social work. The first approach is based on the assumption that a 'profession' could be described in terms of traits (attributes) that are critical to distinguish the 'true' professions from 'occupations'. The widely known definition of profession by Greenwood (1957) contained five such 'critical' attributes: a systematic body of knowledge, publicly recognised authority, community sanction, regulatory code of ethics and professional culture (Weiss-Gal and Welbourne, 2008, p 282). The attributional approach, although criticised for its ahistorical 'naturalism' and functionalistic simplicity, modified by the scholars unsatisfied with the criteria proposed by Greenwood, is still used in numerous studies of professionalisation of social work in different countries (Abbott, 1988; Weiss-Gal and Welbourne, 2008).

The second approach, sometimes called the 'power or control approach', emerged from critical discussions in sociology at the turn of the 1960 and 1970s (Johnson, 1972; Larson, 1977; Abbott, 1988). One of the representatives of this approach is Andrew Abbott, who, in his book The system of professions (1988), proposed an alternative theory of professionalisation in the western world. Abbott's general assumption is that:

> The central phenomenon of professional life is [thus] the link between a profession and its work, a link I shall call jurisdiction. To analyze professional development is to analyze how this link is created in work, how it anchored by formal and informal social structure and the interplay of jurisdictional links between professions determines the history of the individual professions themselves.' (Abbott, 1988, p 20)

Abbott's system model stresses the interdependence of professional development, which reverses the traditional approach to the study of professionalization. This new model, Abbott wrote, 'makes the internal structure of professions one among many determinants of jurisdictional contests and system position … differentiates and conceptualises the various mechanisms through which external social forces affect professions' (Abbott, 1988, p 90). One of these mechanism is 'vacancy creation or abolition but also … changes in the locus of competition (e.g. the dominance of competition in the public or legal-state arenas) and the public criteria of efficacy and legitimacy. External changes may also favour or hinder monopoly and oligopoly in interprofessional relations, affecting the packing of professions into the space of tasks' (Abbott, 1988, p 90).

In this chapter we combine the two approaches presented above – the attributional approach and Abbott's model. Since the state in Poland, like in many other European countries, is a very powerful agent in shaping professions and their jurisdictions, we are going to start with a brief description of the development of social work education and the formation of social work as a separate academic field. Then we will focus on the transformations of the legal and institutional frames of social work practice in the public and private sector after 1989.

The description of professionalisation of social work in Poland is based mainly on our personal experience as academics involved in social work education and training, and participation in preparing and implementing new curricula in social work at the university level from the early 1990s. In addition, we refer to the results of recent studies of professional social work in Poland (Dudkiewicz, 2011; Rymsza, 2011; Kaźmierczak, 2012; Wódz, 2013).

Social work in Poland before and after 1989: historical heritage and the new political reality

The origins of social work in Poland date back to the 1920s and are clearly related to the activities of Helena Radlińska,[2] the founder of the first school for social and educational workers in Warsaw (Studium Pracy Społeczno-Oświatowej in 1925, see: Lepalczyk, 2001). After the Second World War, for political reasons social work in Poland did not win a level of recognition comparable with that in western countries – Great Britain, Sweden or the US. Only in the late 1950s and 1960s did the rebuilding of social services begin, although in a very limited form; the function of the social worker was restored, and the first school for social workers was launched. In 1966 the profession of social assistant appeared in the ministerial list of professions, which allowed training to begin in medical colleges (having the status of high school). The formation of the institutional foundations of social assistance since the late 1960s has been heading toward the creation of local social services, which were functionally linked to healthcare (Oleszczyńska, 1978). In 1975 the majority of social workers were incorporated into the framework of healthcare as workers in social services departments, which were on the margins of healthcare, and they had no chance of any independent action. No legislative regulations in the field of social assistance stated that providing assistance depended largely on the decision of the state administration (the Ministry of Health), which had adequate funds for this purpose. The discretionary nature of social assistance benefits, the lack of guarantees, clients' ability to assert their rights, and organisational and personnel weaknesses, meant that social work did not meet expectations of the concerned populations (Kaźmierczak, 2012).

The actual changes in the development of social work and the social work profession took place just after the political transformation of 1989, in the process of decentralisation of power and the development of local self-government. Thanks to the Social Welfare Act of 1990, social assistance gained importance as a vital area of state social policy, and social work was officially included in the list of mandatory forms of assistance implemented by local governments. The process of professionalisation of social work also accelerated through the development of education, not only at the secondary level, but also at the higher level (at universities and other institutions of higher education).

Referring to the traditional attributional model of professionalisation, we would like to stress that despite efforts in this direction since 1990, the process of professionalisation of social work is still characterised by many shortcomings and weaknesses. Although it has officially been recognised as a profession in its own right (mentioned in the classification of professions since 1966), and since 1990, has had the nature of a regulated profession, it is still not entirely clear what social work is and what it should do within the social welfare system. There is an ongoing discussion about the theoretical foundation of professional practice – to what extent should it draw from other areas of science (pedagogy, sociology, psychology), and to what extent should it create its own distinct scientific basis?

Changing political reality and the locus of the social assistance system in the social policy system have significantly influenced the organisational structure in which social workers operate as well as accompanying standards of education. Due to the assignment of social work activities primarily to public institutions (social welfare centres in the structure of the local government), social workers perform, to a very large extent, administrative and bureaucratic tasks, which significantly limits their ability to pursue social work understood as a methodological activity based on professional knowledge and professional skills. At the same time, as a result of strict regulations controlling access to the profession, social workers have become almost exclusive dispensers of professional social work.

As a result, social workers have fairly limited opportunities to make decisions related to work on the basis of their professional knowledge, skills and values. The ongoing changes related to the standardisation of quality of service of social welfare institutions in practice tend to reduce these possibilities further.

The years 1990-2004 were also marked by very dynamic but chaotic development of educational programmes for social workers both at the level of secondary education and at the level of higher education. At the secondary education level, Social Service Workers Colleges were created, giving license to practise the profession; at higher education institutions, specialisations in social work appeared in various fields (mainly education and sociology), also leading to professional certification.

In the second half of the 1990s, regulations emanating from the Ministry of Labour and Social Policy introduced first- and second-degree qualifications for professional specialisation for social workers and specialists in social service organisations, mandatory for all managers of all institutions in this system. The detailed requirements and minimum curriculum were defined for all providers of education and specialised training. In 2006, social work gained the status of an independent field of study at Bachelor's level, and, in 2011, at Master's level.

During this period, there were also attempts at self-organisation of the environment of social workers. The Polish Association of Social Workers (PTPS) was established, and prepared a draft law on the profession of social worker, but it did not gain recognition in the eyes of experts and representatives of the authorities or among representatives of a large part of the social worker community. The PTPS today plays no role in the integration of social workers into social services organisations or in building the prestige of the profession. However, PTPS's unquestionable achievement is the Code of Ethics of 1998, which was created on the basis of similar documents existing in western countries. Elements of the code are contained in the Social Assistance Act of 2004, but, as research shows, it is not a document widely present in the daily practice of social workers (Dudkiewicz, 2011; Rymsza, 2012).

It is also worth mentioning that the social work profession is quite low on the scale of prestige of professions in Poland, which is undoubtedly related to the low level of remuneration, significantly lower than the salaries of other groups of government workers.

Europeanisation of social welfare in Poland or the paradoxes of top-down modernisation of social work

The analysis of changes in Poland after 1989 indicates that it is interesting to look at the development of the social work profession through the model proposed by Abbott, in which the essence of the professionalisation process is the work performed, not its organisation, and above all the functioning of the profession in a complex system of internal and external dependencies (Abbott 1988).

In the process of professionalisation of social work in Poland there are three main actors: social workers themselves; representatives of the academic community, who since the 1990s have consistently introduced methodical social work into Polish academic research and education as well as into the social assistance system; and representatives of the central administration, who have primarily focused on the creation of legal and organisational regulations regarding social work. Our experience as participants in this process from its beginning is that the role of the third, institutional actor, has increased. In principle, this has not been negative; in some sense it could be perceived as 'natural' in terms of progressing institutionalisation. However, we would like to discuss some of the potentially negative aspects of this increased focus on the institutional actor that we have experienced.

As time goes by, especially in relation to the ongoing process of decentralisation of the state and the dominance of neoliberal rhetoric in the official political discourse, it seems clear that the intention of the government is to monopolise the discourse and limit the impact on it from both experts and academics as well as social workers. A good example is the fact that while new fields of education within the scope of social work have been created, the functions of supervision over the content and certification of training have been entrusted to the Central Examination Commission appointed by the Ministry of Labour and Social Policy. In this way, the government administration obtained a privileged position, at the expense of academics and social workers, in the system of creating and controlling the standards of education for social work in Poland.

The analysis of the formation and changes in regulation of the legal and organisational issues related to social work indicates that we are dealing with the instrumentalisation of the role of academic community, in accordance with the interests of central government (represented by the Ministry of Labour and Social Policy). State monopoly practices escalated especially after 2004, in connection with Poland's accession to the European Union and access to significant financial resources under the EU structural funds. These trends increased even more in the years 2007-13, in connection with the implementation of the Operational Programme of Human Capital Development (financed from the European Social Fund), in which huge funds were allocated to programmes supporting the development of active forms of assistance and support for groups at highest risk of social exclusion (mainly unemployed and disabled people), as well as training and education of social workers. Both social workers and representatives of academic circles have been largely barred from making decisions on the merits of this programme, as well as organisational issues. It is significant, as studies show, that a policy of 'activation' – introduced 10 years ago at the level of statutory regulation – has had little effect on changing the model of social services 'at the bottom', where a clerical approach is still dominant and only corresponds to a small extent to the requirements of professional action (Dudkiewicz, 2011).

The last amendment to the Social Assistance Act, which was set to be implemented during 2015, proposed several changes to the current shape of the social assistance system (Ministry of Labour and Social Policy, 2014). These changes were not implemented by the new Government, created by PiS (Law and Justice) who came to power after the parliamentary elections in Autumn 2015. From the very start, it calls for the intensification of social work activities, inter alia by giving priority to preventive measures, activation policies and social services, to provide opportunities specifically for professional social workers. However, further reading of the draft amendments raises doubts as to whether this is the case. It is worth mentioning three of important elements in this regard.

First, according to the logic of New Public Management, as previously mentioned, it is the intention, to a much greater extent than has hitherto been the case, to allow non-state actors (both social and private) to act as social service agencies. As stated in the draft amendments:

> Inter alia, NGOs, institutions defined in regulations on social employment and social cooperatives, will be able to obtain the Status of Social Services Agency. Entities founded by natural persons, having necessary professional qualifications (e.g. social workers), conducting jointly their business activity may also request the status of agency. (Ministry of Labour and Social Policy, 2014, p 18)

One of the requirements for obtaining such status is to have a minimum of two social workers at the agency's disposal, preferably with certain specialisations. Therefore, there is no unambiguously defined requirement for the social services agency to employ social workers; 'having at one's disposal' may, in fact, mean that social workers will be used to perform tasks unrelated to their profession, and the need for specialist qualifications is only 'advisable'. In cases where a social service agency is assigned work covering a large number of clients, the requisite number of two social workers is bound to be insufficient, meaning that some activities of a social nature would have to be carried out by personnel with no relevant qualifications.

The second issue concerns social work in social assistance centres. On the one hand, it is planned that social work will be radically separated from the administration of benefits, in line with the express wishes of large numbers of social workers. The intention is to release social workers from administrative and bureaucratic activities, leaving social work as their only duty. At the same time, however, we do not find any specification in the amendments concerning the definition of such social work and how it should be executed. Therefore, the social workers are left without a clear formulation of their duties, which means there is a lack of unambiguous criteria for accounting for and assessing their work. The wording relating to the conduct of social work, which has been adopted in the postulated new tasks of social assistance centres at the municipal level, is based on medical history and social contracts; it is clearly restrictive and does not go beyond the scope of current practice. It is also worth noting that conducting social work was not mentioned among the proposed new tasks of social assistance institutions at the level of powiat[3] (Powiat Centre for Family Support).

In addition, it is proposed that in the field of prevention services for individuals and families, which will be provided as part of social work, a social worker will provide preventive social support for individuals and families – that is, act as a social assistant. This raises the question of whether social assistants will come into conflict with family assistants, whose duties are worded in a similar way. Under the Support for the Family and the Foster Care Act (Journal of Laws No. 149/2011, item 887) such a function may be performed by persons without licences and qualifications to carry out the social work. In addition, the work that family assistants do cannot be combined with social worker duties, and they do not have to be employed in social welfare centres.

In light of the above, the attempt by neighbouring care services to expand the directory of services seems but a trifle. The way in which the formalisation of this service is envisaged is an example of how the right idea can have the opposite effect.

The third issue deserving attention is the intention to incorporate social services standards into the social assistance system.

Standardisation of social services in Poland and its possible consequences for the social work profession

Over the past several years, there has been a significant change in attitude towards the social security system in Poland, including the social welfare system. Signs of this include the commercialisation of public social welfare through the use of management models developed in the market sector (TQM, ISO 9901) (Kowalczyk and Krzyszkowski, 2011; Krzyszkowski, no date), the implementation of formal control procedures (largely in connection with the implementation of projects financed by the European Social Fund), and the promotion of ideas of social work in terms of standardised services, which lends itself to formalised procedures and criteria of evaluation (Szarfenberg, 2011). Excessive standardisation of social work is, in our opinion, erroneous and contrary to the very essence of social work. It is a misconception to promote the system projects in POKL (in which opportunities to present alternatives are limited) involving one pattern or model of work with different categories of customers, communities, and so forth. The analysis of the content of these standards, developed in a manner that in itself raises many doubts,[4] shows that in large part they coincide with the scope of professional knowledge, skills and competences acquired during the education and training for social workers.

The unavoidable question therefore is what is the point of setting up such standards? Imposing one standard of service is questionable, when the desire for individualisation and the strengthening of client subjectivity, aid schemes and support systems has been declared. Clients should have greater responsibility for overcoming their problems, which has been the case to date, for example by the conscious selection of solutions that have been offered to them. Professionally trained social workers, with competence in methodical social work, should constitute a sufficient guarantee of compliance with the standards of assistance intervention, regardless of their employer institution. The only requirement is to be well educated and have adequate opportunities for professional development.

In addition, these standards are developed in a way that does not take into account the reality of the Polish social assistance system. Most of the social assistance centres operating in the small municipalities, as well as other institutions and organisations dealing with social issues, will not be able to meet them for a very prosaic reason – they do not have, and probably will not have soon at their disposal, sufficiently large numbers of specialised staff, including social workers, able to fulfil all the requirements of the standards. Even if we take into account the new requirement for increasing social worker provision per head of population,[5] it will not have much impact on the burden of duties imposed on social workers. In conjunction with the lack of a clear definition of what social work ought to involve, it is tantamount to tacit approval for small social assistance centres to focus on formal rather than on merit-related activities – in other words, to continue with the status quo.

It should be stressed that in Poland, unlike in other countries, there is little requirement in standards for social services provision for upholding users' rights (Lafore and Borgetto, 2000).

To sum up, we can say that we are dealing on the one hand with a sort of recentralisation of the social assistance system, and on the other hand, with an attempt to get rid of the responsibility for carrying out social work tasks effectively. Because the state (central administration) is increasingly putting itself in the role of sole oracle of what is right, proper and adequate, it thereby demonstrates a lack of confidence in the people who create the social assistance system (that is, social workers and the broadly understood academic community). At the same time, the state reinforces the role of non-professional, third-sector agents in the provision of social services tasks, hitherto reserved principally for professional social workers. It also tries to shift the responsibility for implemented measures to external actors. At the same time, it attempts to retain, and even increase, its influence and control over social work provision through the enormous financial resources at its disposal, namely funds from the European Union under the Financial Perspectives 2014-20 initiative.

Conclusion

If we look at the recent development of the social work profession in Poland by using Abbott's concept of professionalisation of social work as the 'interplay between the internal structure of professions and external social forces which affect the professions', we may say that professional practice was, and still is, shaped mainly by state regulations, sometimes very restrictive and contradictory, with negative consequences for the social worker's professional autonomy. The excessive state regulation and control of professional practice is not counter-balanced by the activities performed by the social workers themselves or by other actors within academia. Social workers are failing to oppose state regulation because of weaknesses in professional self-organisation. Actors within academia are failing to oppose it due to the lack of consensus regarding fundamental questions, such as the necessity to develop social work as a separate academic field and the legitimacy of the old and new social professions (social pedagogues, psychologists, socio-therapists, street workers, social animators, family and old/disabled persons assistants, and so on) to fulfil social work tasks. This situation is clearly not favourable for the strengthening of the professional identity of social workers in the future. A more optimistic scenario is possible, however, if social workers themselves assume a more active attitude towards the preservation of professional standards and the development of professional culture. The academic community has also a positive role to play by making continuous efforts to legitimise the profession through data-driven discussions among supporters of different approaches and schools of social work.

Notes

1 A mature profession is defined by its specific function in society and by a set of traits attributed to professions by scholars like Greenwood (1957) and his followers.

[2] Helena Radlińska (1879-1954) was the founder of social pedagogy in Poland, an activist of the patriotic movement for the popular education, a scientist and the author of many books and papers fundamental for the development of the innovative pedagogical thought at the turn of the 19th and the 20th centuries in Poland. Studium Pracy Społeczno- Oświatowej (Social and Educational Work Study Centre), opened by Helena Radlińska in 1925 in Warsaw, was the first attempt towards the formal education of social workers in Poland. Radlińska's original theory of social work, understood as a conscious educational activity, oriented towards the transformation of human environment by people who create this environment themselves, is still considered as the basis for the formation of social work in Poland. For more see: Lepalczyk, 2001.

[3] Powiat is a territorial administrative unit in Poland (intermediary between the level of municipality and county).

[4] These standards were developed in a project implemented by non-governmental organizations in partnership with the Ministry of Labour and Social Policy. Reading these undoubtedly interesting materials leaves quite an ambivalent impression; on the one hand, it shows the immensity of the work done within only a few years by a relatively small group of experts involved in the project, on the other, it makes one reflect on the accuracy of the selected 'path' for modernising social services, implemented according to formulas developed not during an open public debate, but among selected experts invited to implement system projects (Wódz, 2013).

[5] Currently the Social Welfare Act imposes on social assistance centres an obligation to employ one social worker per 2,000 inhabitants; according to the new provision, there should be one social worker per 50 families/cases.

References

Abbott, A. (1988) *The system of professions. An essay on the division of expert labor*, Chicago, IL: University of Chicago Press.

Abbott, A. (1995) 'Boundaries of social work or social work of boundaries?', *Social Service Review*, 69: 545-62.

Dudkiewicz, M. (ed) (2011) *Pracownicy socjalni: Pomiędzy instytucją pomocy społecznej a środowiskiem lokalnym* [Social workers: Between welfare institution and the local environment], Warszawa: Instytut Spraw Publicznych.

Flexner, A. (1915) 'Is social work a profession?', National Conference of Charities and Corrections, *Proceedings of the National Conference of Charities and Corrections at the forty-second annual session held in Baltimore, Maryland, May 12-19,* Chicago, IL: Hildmann.

Greenwood, E. (1957) 'Attributes of a profession', *Social Work*, 2: 65-74.

Johnson, T. (1972) *Professions and power*, London: Macmillan.

Kaźmierczak, T. (2012) 'W cieniu prawa ubogich: o źródłach i rozwoju (praktykowanej w OPS) pracy socjalnej' [In the shadow of the rights of the poor: and the sources of development (as practiced in OPS) of social work], in T. Kaźmierczak and M. Rymsza (eds) *W stronę aktywnych służb społecznych* [Towards active social services], Warszawa: Instytut Spraw Publicznych and Centrum Aaktywności Lokalnej, pp 109-32.

Kowalczyk, B. and Krzyszkowski, J. (2011) 'Modele sposobu realizacji usług o określonym standardzie w jednostkach organizacyjnych pomocy i integracji społecznej' [Models of how to implement services of a certain standard in organisational units of social assistance and integration], in R. Szarfenberg (ed) *Krajowy Raport Badawczy. Pomoc i integracja społeczna wobec wybranych grup – diagnoza standaryzacji usług i modeli instytucji* [National Research Report. Assistance and social integration of selected groups – diagnosis of standardization of services and institutional models], Warszawa: WRZOS.

Krzyszkowski, J. (no date) *Nowe zarządzanie (menadżerskie lub partycypacyjne) instytucjami pomocy społecznej. Systemy zarządzania jakością ISO w instytucjach pomocy społecznej, Ekspertyza w ramach projektu 1.18: Tworzenie i rozwijanie standardów usług pomocy i integracji społecznej*' [New management (managerial or participatory) in social welfare institutions. ISO quality management systems in the institutions of social welfare, Expertise in the framework of the system project 1.18 'Creating and developing standards of assistance and social integration'], Warszawa: Centrum Rozwoju Zasobów Ludzkich.

Lafore, R. and Borgetto, M. (2000) *La République sociale. Contribution à l'étude de la question démocratique en France* [The social Republic. Contribution to the study of the question of democracy in France], Paris: PUF.

Larson, M.S. (1977) *The rise of professionalism*, Berkeley, CA: University of California Press.

Lepalczyk, I. (2001) *Helena Radlińska* - życie i twórczość [Helena Radlińska – life and work], Toruń: Wydawnictwo Adam Marszałek.

Ministry of Labour and Social Policy (2014) Projekt założeń projektu ustawy o zmianie ustawy o pomocy społecznej oraz niektórych innych ustaw. Wariant II, sierpień 2014 [The draft of guidelines for amending the law on social assistance and certain other laws. Option II, August 2014], Warszawa: Ministerstwo Pracy i Polityki Społecznej.

Oleszczyńska, A. (1978) *Pracownik socjalny w pomocy społecznej* [Social worker in social services], Warszawa: Instytut Wydawniczy CRZZ.

Program Operacyjny Kapitał Ludzki 2007-2013 [Human Capital Operational Programme 2007-2013], Warszawa: Ministerstwo Rozwoju Regionalnego.

Rymsza, M. (ed) (2011) *Czy podejście aktywizujące ma szansę?* [Has activation approached a chance?], Warszawa: Instytut Spraw Publicznych.

Rymsza, M. (ed) (2012) *Pracownicy socjalni i praca socjalna w Polsce. Między służbą a urzędem* [Social workers and social work in Poland. Between social service and administration], Warszawa: Instytut Spraw Publicznych.

Szarfenberg, R. (2011) 'Standardy i standaryzacja pracy socjalnej i usług pomocy i integracji społecznej' [Standards and standardization of social services, social assistance and integration], in R. Szarfenberg (ed) *Krajowy Raport Badawczy. Pomoc i integracja społeczna wobec wybranych grup – diagnoza standaryzacji usług i modeli instytucji* [National Research Report. Assistance and social integration of selected groups – diagnosis of standardization of services and institutional models], Warszawa: WRZOS.

Weiss-Gal, I. and Welbourne, P. (2008) 'The professionalisation of social work: a cross-national exploration', *International Journal of Social Welfare*, 17(4): 281-90.

Wenocur, S. and Reisch, M. (1983) 'The social work profession and the ideology of professionalization', *Journal of Sociology and Social Welfare*, 10: 684-732.

Wódz, K. (2013) *Instytucjonalne bariery rozwoju środowiskowej metody pracy socjalnej/organizowania społeczności lokalnej w Polsce. Ekspertyza przygotowana dla Instytutu Spraw Publicznych w ramach projektu systemowego 1.18: 'Tworzenie i rozwijanie standardów usług pomocy i integracji społecznej'* [Institutional barriers to the development of environmental methods in social work/community organization in Poland. Expertise prepared for the Institute of Public Affairs in the framework of the system project 1.18 'Creating and developing standards of assistance and social integration'], Warszawa: Instytut Spraw Publicznych.

Part 3
Collaboration, conflict and competition

EIGHT

Professional boundary crossing and interprofessional knowledge development

Ilse Julkunen and Elisabeth Willumsen

Introduction

A significant trait of modern societies is the increased organisational specialisation of welfare services, which in turn has resulted in increased professionalisation, that is, a greater number of professionals involved in the production of welfare services (Meads and Ashcroft, 2005). This growing specialisation and professionalisation, which on one hand has led to more advanced services, has also resulted in fragmentation and need for coordination between services in order to provide adequate and holistic efforts when responding to service users' complex needs (Arnkil and Seikkula, 2015). Today the service delivery system is faced with problems concerning the division of labour, coordination of services, maintenance and development of staff competence, and improvement of service effectiveness and outcomes. Specialisation often necessitates collaboration between different actors in order to achieve a comprehensive view of citizens' complex problems.

The aim of this chapter is to examine how interprofessional knowledge is developed when crossing boundaries, illustrated by two cases in social work in the domain of child welfare in Norway and Finland. We have chosen these two cases to provide analytic description of innovative knowledge production processes in professional practices and the complex boundary crossings involved. The two cases represent the field of child and youth welfare, a field that is under much pressure both on a national and on an international level.

Interprofessional practices

There is an obvious need for developing multi- or interprofessional services that address complex problems effectively. By way of example, doctors, social workers and other welfare professionals in the welfare services need to find new ways of collaborating to be able to solve complex cases. To ensure optimal outcomes for service users in an uncertain, evolving environment, it is necessary to enhance professional knowledge and skills in boundary crossing and increase efforts to adapt to change. These challenges certainly involve European welfare states and highlight the ultimate purpose: 'to assure universal coverage of high quality comprehensive services that are essential to advance opportunity for health equity within and between countries' (Frenk et al, 2010), mentioning improved team work and decreased professional tribalism as important issues.

It is claimed that the prevalence of difficulties of children and young people is high, and that 15-20% of all children have psychiatric problems that influence their level of functioning (NOU, 2009, p 18). International research show that serious behavioural problems ('conduct disorder') comprise 1.5-3.4 % of all children (five times as many boys than girls) (Barton and Parry-Jones, 2004, p 1632). No matter which numbers are utilised and which problems identified, child and youth welfare is characterised by uncertainty, complexity and unpredictability. Hence, a significant number of children will need interprofessional provision and support in an attempt to prevent serious problems for children at risk and their families as well as to limit the need for increasing resources in a long-term perspective.

Our interest in these cases is to examine the boundary activities in knowledge development of interprofessional practices. Interprofessional practices imply complex networks of relationships and they go beyond the more contemporary forms of coordination and thus form an interesting ground for managing and creating knowledge across boundaries. The first case, on initial collaboration with young people at risk, is a Finnish research and development project where different professionals from various sectors conceptualise their role, and the help and support given to young people at risk, and form a model aimed at improving the initial collaboration practices. The other case, concerning young children with attention deficit hyperactivity disorder (ADHD)/Asperger syndrome, is a Norwegian research and development project that focuses on how professionals discuss their conception and responsibilities in dealing with families and children in need for the purpose of improving services and facilitating organisational change. Both these projects serve as examples of crossing boundaries and reflect the growing need of developing interprofessional practices and achieving knowledge about how these processes develop over time. A transitional framework, developed by Michel Callon

(1986), is used for the analysis. He developed this framework while studying the anchorage of scallops in the Mediterranean area, a framework that was retrospectively (and inductively) created on basis of different sorts of meetings and exchanges (including negotiations), and adjustments among the actors in the case study. He found that four key questions needed to be addressed in order to scrutinise the elements of the complex process. The first concerns problematisation: it is important identify the issue and phenomenon that require a solution and to ask how the problem is identified by the different actors. The second concerns the degree to which the different actors are invested in the solution to the issue and how they conceptualise their roles and responsibilities. The third focuses on visions. Here it is crucial to analyse how the different actors see their role in a new setting, and how they can be encouraged to change and create new visions. The fourth concerns the anchorage of new working models and the types of ally mobilised. Although the framework as such has not been developed within the context of interprofessional practices but within that of scientific research, it is applicable to other settings (Star and Griesemer, 1989) and provides a tool for structuring and pinpointing the places and phases where boundary activities are formed. It also helps with focusing on which boundary activities are important for the development of shared knowledge and where critical pitfalls may be found. Wenger's concept of community of practice (Wenger, 1998) serves further as an analytical approach to analyse more deeply the multilateral and dynamic boundaries in how professionals may or may not/can or cannot/choose or choose not to cross professional boarders in order to attend to the mutual project of the community of practice. Hence, the concept of community of practice goes beyond professional boundaries and analyses how the professionals in the projects cross boundaries in order to create interfaces for collaboration and knowledge development.

Collaborative practice and boundary crossings

In the literature on interprofessional collaborative practice there is still some confusion surrounding the motivations behind this process as well as the definitions used. The processes of specialisation, professionalisation and fragmentation are part of the societal development framing the welfare services, both nationally and internationally, and there has been a demand for collaboration over the past 25 years (Barr et al, 2005). Abbott (1988) reminds us that these processes are also involved in framing the professional jurisdiction, that is, the link between a profession and its work regarding professional control over knowledge and skills connected to tasks and contexts. But the same conditions that necessitate collaboration can also hamper interaction because of demarcation problems and competition between different professions – so-called professional tribalism. Even though the focus has been on collaboration for a long time, it seems that there is great confusion in the use of terms of interprofessional collaboration and little empirical evidence for the efficacy of interprofessional work or for how interprofessional knowledge is being developed in boundary-crossing practices. As Seaburn and colleagues (1996, p 23) have noted, 'A culture of collaboration does not just happen. It must be formed and fashioned by many hands.'

The World Health Organization's *Framework for action on interprofessional education and collaborative practice* (WHO, 2010) defines collaboration as follows: 'Collaborative practice happens when multiple health workers from different professional backgrounds work together with patients, families, carers and communities to deliver the highest quality of care (p 7)'. This comes close to Payne's definition of 'the open team' (2000), 'the professional and multiprofessional teams and the network of people we link with in the community and teamworking and networking as an integrated form of practice' (p 5). The definition allows for inclusion of professionals and service users, as well as organisations such as agencies and units/departments. It also focuses on the main desirable outcome of collaboration – an *integrated practice*. The importance of integration lies in its capacity to relate to the demands of the environment and to meet people's multiple needs, that is, those of various target groups for social work, such as children and families. The term 'open team' indicates that the team's boundaries are transparent and blurred, in order to allow the members to adapt to the situation of the service user, the development of his/her situation, the need for changing competence and services and so on. All in all, the definition attends to the complex and dynamic interaction between various actors and services and moreover the collaboration process.

The very idea and language of interprofessional practice implies boundaries. These complex networks of relationships offer different possibilities for thinking about self and others. When talking about interprofessionalism, Abbott (1988) sees boundaries as closed doors, claiming that professionals struggle and compete for maintaining jurisdiction and distribution of tasks and that this is a way of controlling professional knowledge and hence creating boundaries for exclusion. Wheatley (2005), on the other hand, sees boundaries as places of meeting and exchange rather than a self-protective wall. We usually think of boundaries as the means to define separateness, defining what is inside or what is outside. But in living systems, boundaries are quite different. They can be the places where new relationships take form, exchange and grow. This is also well illuminated in the Callon's case study on the anchorage of scallops and what he observed during the process. Similarly, Wenger (1998) looks at boundaries multilaterally; boundaries may serve as sources for misunderstandings, disagreements and conflicts causing communication problems, but may also be viewed as interfaces for contact and interaction that may promote coordination, in other words spaces for integration and knowledge development. Hence, boundaries represent places where collaboration may be created and organised and may have the potential for hampering as well as supporting coordination, knowledge development and change. Concepts have been developed to more thoroughly explicate the multidimensionality of boundary crossing, such as boundary practices (Wenger, 1998), boundary objects (Star and Griesemer, 1989; Wenger, 1998), and knowledge managing across boundaries (Carlile, 2004), as which we shall discuss further.

Examining collaborative practices in social work

In looking at the boundary crossings of interprofessional collaboration, we provide an analytical description of two case studies of knowledge development processes applying Callon's (1986) framework. We have both been involved in these case studies as researchers and supervisors, and here we attempt retrospectively to capture the spaces and objects that either form barriers or facilitate development.

The case studies

'Systemic work with young people at risk' was a research and development project on how professional groups and organisations deliver help and support to young people at risk and how they together work on ways to improve initial collaboration practices with this group of citizens. The two-year research and development project (Söderström and Backman, 2012) was organised to develop new collaborative working models within a broad network of people from different institutions and professions, such as schools, day care, healthcare, family counselling and child protection. An overarching goal was to develop a service user-oriented, systemic collaboration model with the prevailing structural and organisational forms as it standpoints. This assumed developing knowledge in a dialogic approach and involving frontline practitioners within the development work.

'Together for children and young people' was a research and development project that focused on how professionals understand and discuss their perception and responsibilities in dealing with families and children in need in order to improve services and facilitate organisational change (Elvik and Willumsen, 2011). The project was organised to ensure the goal of coordinated services for children with psychiatric difficulties and behavioural problems such as ADHD/Asperger syndrome. Considerable disagreements regarding responsibility/accountability for this target group, particularly between health and child welfare services, were registered in the municipality. Schools and psychiatric services were involved occasionally when necessary. Although internal procedures existed, these were not sufficient to clarify responsibility in actual cases. The characteristics of this group of young people, close to 18 years of age, were significant psychiatric difficulties and functional disabilities, with implications for parental care and fulfilling school work. Hence, these young people and families' needs were complex and challenging to professionals in terms of understanding their situation and their struggles. In order to work systematically to improve the coordination/integration of services for this target group, an external supervisor was invited to discuss actual cases.

Investment of actors

We were interested in analysing the degree to which relevant actors were invested in solutions to these difficult cases and how they conceptualised their roles and responsibilities. At the start the professionals in the different domains were all overwhelmed by the challenges of the child and youth welfare services and found that there were too many obstacles to finding help and sustainable solutions for young people and their families. Which services were most relevant was an open question, hence causing confusion between social workers from health and child welfare services respectively. Moreover, there was little knowledge on the division of labour, what other professionals' roles and tasks were. For instance, teachers involved in these cases would come into contact with the children in school, but had few dealings with their parents. Their understanding of their role was one of advice without the possibility of intervention, leading to a lot of frustration and also mistrust towards other welfare professionals.

The professionals used quite a bit of time to clarify the primary problem because this would give the direction for which service had to take responsibility. At the same time, the problems were so complex that it was not easy to identify just one. Dealing with young people and their families within conflicting frames caused discussion, confusion, frustration and also power struggles between collaborating partners. The professionals represented health, education and childcare services, and each assumed their own assessment of the young people and their families. From the start, the professionals were caught in different administrative silos, albeit governed by the same municipality. This results in an emphasis on administrative power struggles, which in turn may lead to the avoidance of responsibility. The organisational boundaries seemed thus to form an uncomfortable place. The danger of silos is that they may become isolated from the practices they are supposed to connect (Wenger, 1998; Bihari Axelsson and Axelsson, 2009). This often leads to fragmentation and multi-professional collaboration that implies mechanical coordination with a low degree of integration and the lack of potential for the development of novel interventions (Willumsen, 2009).

Translating meanings may be seen as an externalisation process that adds to addressing differences across the different domains as well as being a prerequisite to learning processes that examine ways of thinking (Nonaka, 1994). But while different interests are often revealed they can also create barriers to developing shared meanings. Callon (1986) focused on dwelling thoroughly on different interests and saw this stage as crucial in arriving to a careful analysis of the problematics at hand. Hence, this stage involves negotiating interests and making trade-offs between actors (Wenger, 1998; Carlile, 2004) and may involve revealing power interests and moving beyond the 'here and now'.

Just initiating collaboration seemed a mountainous effort for the professionals and almost an impossible task. Emotional elements played a key role in discussing these issues, and either facilitated or inhibited collaboration. Interestingly, the professionals described the problematics of collaboration as 'out there', as something that was not concretely contained by the professionals themselves. In acknowledging the emotional and practical experiences of professionals, Strauss (1993) pointed out the importance of interaction at every level, ranging from the most collective to the most individual. This relationship between the individual and the collective is also a crucial building block to open up for broader visions of change.

As long as professionals suggest what others should do, and resist committing to and taking responsibility, they keep themselves out of the collaboration process. Arnkil and Seikkula (2015) claim that it is when professionals see themselves as part of the hopelessness that they can begin to see the process from a personal perspective. Taking the position of an outsider prevents one from looking for plausible solutions. Solutions are often 'smaller' and simpler than when looking from an outside position. The systemic perspective was pervasive in the Finnish case and encompassed a view that changes in the system are possible through changing one's own behaviour and thinking.

To deal with processes with different interests implies identifying boundary objects, objects that are 'common enough to more than one world to make them recognisable' (Star and Griesemer, 1989, p 393). Carlile (2004) points out that under these circumstances domain-specific knowledge may need to be translated and transformed to effectively share and assess knowledge at the boundary. Hence, the central collaborative task is the translation of each other's perspectives.

Working with difficult issues

When analysing a complex and dynamic field, such as interprofessional collaboration, it is important to acknowledge the process and the length of time as well as the different levels involved. These comprise the personal level (professionals and service users participating in collaboration), and organisational the level, for example, organisations, units and sections. We were interested in looking at how professionals created opportunities and how they worked with difficult issues.

Ways of dealing with problematic issues were facilitated through regular working seminars and learning forums led by supervisors. The working seminars were planned collaboratively with actors and project leaders. They covered theoretical knowledge on interprofessional collaboration, systemic approaches, dialogic methods and user perspectives. Learning forums were created to provide support for testing new ideas for pilot units and the networks around them. Because of the different organisational settings of the cases involved, these learning fora were different. The Finnish project focused on border-crossing learning forums, whereas the Norwegian project aimed to create a 'learning organisation' to facilitate systematised improvements and implementation in the municipality as a whole. In the community of practice approach, these could be seen as boarder activities and boarder objects, including different levels of learning, personal, collective and peripheral learning. The Finnish case had different learning forums for the professionals involved, with a professional group leader functioning as a moderator. The moderator helped the group to deliberate on their own positions and occupational roles.

Both of the projects built their reflections on concrete and challenging client cases. In the Norwegian case, the supervision meetings started with the presentation of a client case. During these reflections, the participants could explain, elaborate on and examine nuances in their views, ask questions and clarify their thoughts and perceptions. There was also a focus on clarifying roles and responsibilities. In the Finnish case, there was in the beginning a resistance to discussing challenging cases openly and in participating in developing new forms of collaboration. A lot of work was needed to create and manage boundary objects. One essential element in the process was the translation of each other's perspectives. Star and Griesemer (1989) claim that the central cooperative task of social worlds is a key process in developing and maintaining coherence across intersecting worlds. Translation needs to include learning phases. This was made possible through a learning model based on critical reflection of client cases developed by Ray Pawson (2008). This systemic and reflective model helped with the acknowledgement and acceptance of the different roles and responsibilities of each professional. It also encouraged a commitment to developing a new working model.

The peripheral learning elements were made possible through seminars for members of the project team and other interested persons in the municipality, including plenary sessions on relevant topics and interprofessional group discussions. The supervisor in the Norwegian project was responsible for a presentation on the theory of collaboration in seminars, which constituted a mutual framework for the supervision meetings. In the Finnish case, the issues and themes were driven by the needs of the units and their networks and were based on the concrete and daily experiences of the professionals. In the Norwegian case, the supervisor had a strong translator and gatekeeper role. She took part in supervision meetings at the health and social centres and participated in the project group at an administrative level. She provided information on activities and progress and pointed out areas for improvement. She also presented written information summarising points for improvement to be discussed by the project group, which were followed up by the project management and extended to other parts of the organisation/municipality. Some of the 'improvement points' were introduced as main topics for mutual discussion at the seminars.

In the beginning there seemed to be a lack of communication between the partners due to the absence of a common framework.

Much work was made on creating boundary objects. In everyday life, we constantly deal with artefacts that connect us in various ways to practices we do or do not belong to, claims Wenger (1998). It seemed that the 'not-knowing' element in both projects produced a boundary that both shut and opened doors. Opening these doors leads to more than just information transmission – in both cases, partners worked intensively on dialogues and reflection, allowing space for experiences and values, and thus creating a sense of a shared belonging. Bhaskar and Danermark (2006) point out in their work on interdisciplinary collaboration that meaning is formed through interactive communication. This includes being open to conflicting discussions, just as Callon points out. This was well illustrated in the reflective discussions in both cases with room for thought and talk that allowed for transformations in ways of understanding context.

What type of boundary crossing was taking place?

Establishing boundary practices

In both projects there was an urge to improve services and develop new forms/models of collaboration to integrate efforts more efficiently. Both projects were establishing boundary practices (Wenger, 1998), that is, organising fora and meeting places for mutual engagement, building and maintaining relationships between insiders and outsiders and developing a repertoire to address conflicts, reconcile perspectives and approaches and find resolutions. Such boundary practices may over time develop a community of practice that goes beyond administrative and professional boundaries, in order to engage in productive activities that imply negotiating diverging meanings and approaches, such as in collaborative work with children and families.

One example from the Norwegian case concerned a family with multiple problems where the professionals from municipality and psychiatric units were frustrated and felt that team meetings were a waste of time. The case coordinator wanted to discuss the family in the supervision meeting and it was decided to organise the following team meeting as part of the supervision process. This was a way of establishing a boundary practice whereby all the professionals involved could participate in mutual reflections. The coordinator conducted the meeting as usual, and the supervisor was allowed to interrupt and reformulate questions and ask for elaborations. The meeting turned out to be a 'live' performance of communication and problem solving, where the participants had the opportunity to explain and give reasons for their perceptions and actions. Several questions were clarified and a plan for follow-up was agreed, resulting in a positive outcome for the family. The professionals thought they had learned from each other, were able to give each other positive feedback and commented that the family had been kept in centre of the discussion. Hence, the combination of reflection and establishing a boundary practice turned out to be fruitful. In the long term, it is important to encourage the establishment of boundary practices, because they may serve as starting points for tailoring combinations of services for particular service users. Additionally, members develop a repertoire of knowledge and skills when they share their knowledge, in terms of assessing each other's domain-specific knowledge as well as developing common knowledge to better understand the challenges they face when trying to work across professional and agency boundaries (Carlile, 2004).

Wenger acknowledges the importance of peripheral experiences. The ability to have multiple levels of involvement is an important characteristic, one that presents opportunities for learning both for outsiders and for communities, claims Wenger (1998, p 117). The projects in our study were both encouraged to communicate with broader networks and the seminars provided space for reflection both outside and inside the communities.

Creating boundary objects

Although boundary practices may serve as spaces for collaborative work, there is no guarantee that collaboration will happen. The participating members may have to create boundary objects, that is, objects that serve to coordinate the perspectives of various constituencies and practices for some purpose (Star and Griesemer, 1989). In most services, boundary objects are already in place, such as mutual records/files, computer systems containing standardised information, manuals and reports. However, these devices may not necessarily ensure specific tasks in collaborative work. For instance, in Scandinavia, the Individual Plan (IP) (Kjellevold, 2013) has been established as a legal framework for the coordination of services and may be regarded as a boundary object. Still, only a small amount of the estimated population has an IP. The reconstruction of the practices during supervision showed us that the creation of additional boundary objects, such as forms/templates for supervision, reports of activities and references to relevant literature, need to be worked on in order to improve communication.

Creating boundary objects may also be regarded as a management tool in order to connect functions and tasks with relevant communities of practice in order to facilitate shared practice. In this sense the boundary object may go beyond professional jurisdictions and require a process of translation between each form of partial jurisdiction (Wenger, 1989). Additionally, the boundary object may go across administrative silos to support mutual initiatives. Both boundary practices and boundary objects influence the participants' attitudes and whether they choose to cross boundaries in order to create interfaces for collaboration and knowledge development.

But boundary objects are not always a question of concrete tools but of shared artefacts. When looking back at the knowledge development process, participants in both of our case studies emphasised trust. Trust was an importance ingredient in the working process and formed an essential boundary object. Trust enabled creativity and courage to try new working forms. Working together on real cases had an impact on the groups at an emotional level. Trust towards others in the group enabled participants to give constructive criticism to others without excluding themselves from the process. The common ground started to take form as common concepts, and terminology enabled boundary crossing. Instead of concentrating on professional boundaries, the object of the practice, the child and the family became important. This gave room for another dynamic in the interaction with the professionals and a new form of knowledge building.

Encouraging boundary spanners

Bridge builders or boundary spanners play a key role in the process of establishing boundary practices and creating boundary objects. According to Wenger (1989), such actors have experience in multiple work practices and are able to transfer some element of one practice to another, also called brokering. The focus is on the relationship between a community of practice and the external environment, across boundaries and between practices, a complex process that include influencing the development of a practice, addressing conflicting interests, facilitating transactions and enabling learning between practices. Boundary spanners demonstrate particular competence in greasing the wheels between professionals and organisations by facilitating dialogue and negotiating goals and meanings regarding inherent conflicts across boundaries (Oliver, 2013).

In our case studies we noticed several examples of boundary spanning. The leaders of the reflective teams, whether supervisors or educators, are perhaps the most evident boundary spanners, although their productivity depends much on communications and negotiations between the different actors. Sometimes these involve power struggles, as with one of the groups in the Finnish case. However, boundary spanners are not only an issue of competencies but of doing, thinking and saying, and these characteristics may differ in different contexts.

One could say that a variety of contributions from professions and organisations are needed, which implies differentiation, as well as the unified efforts necessary to achieve integration. Oliver (2013) emphasises the importance of acknowledging and valuing difference in terms of culture, role and focus. One could say that value creation emerges through experiences and interpretations of values inherent in work practices. All professions have their own ethical values and code of ethics of how to do good practice (Molander and Terum, 2008), but they come alive in practice in collaboration with the user. Hence, values are wedded to actions in practice, and these came to light when the practitioners reflected on real cases. Boundary spanners were often needed to translate this domain-specific knowledge.

Conclusion: readiness for complexity?

The growing trend towards the development of boundary crossing and interprofessional services has been particularly common between the health and social sectors. The aim of this chapter has been to explore how interprofessional knowledge is developed when crossing boundaries, illustrated by two cases in the field of child welfare from Norway and Finland. The chapter points to the necessity to build knowledge development on existing knowledge, routines and values. Sustainable changes are not about 'shaking it all up' or 'turning everything upside down', rather, questions of values are embedded and acted out in concrete situations. Questions about interests and values in professional working life are present when practitioners encounter, and when their values and visions are included in, organisational change processes. Practitioners' values and visions provide guidelines for what may reasonably be changed and what may be preserved. The chapter also acknowledges that practitioners' access to knowledge development processes is vital for both desired change and competence development.

Together these workings are still not enough, as they need to be contextualised, confined and grounded through different organisational and network levels. Change requires organisation-level measures in order to support new working models. Accordingly, practices call for commitment from organisations' management. Knowledge development, however, calls for moving beyond information transmission and management by focusing on the relational dimension and by highlighting reflexive analysis and deliberation about values and interests in practice (see also Nowotny, 2003). The cases scrutinised in this chapter may form an illustrative example on how professionals in the welfare field initiate new ways of working in practice on the basis of their values, and these new ways may contain potential for an extension of being and doing.

Analytically we found it intriguing to use the conceptual framework of community of practice and the interrelations between different boundary concepts, which managed to open up the phenomenon on interprofessional collaboration. We also found Callon's careful (1986) analysis of the problematics at hand as important, as it reveals power interests and may serve as an iterative framework within which actors may assess each other's knowledge.

All in all, we found the approach 'dialectical, emphasising the relationships of each part to each other and to the whole' (Worrall, 2010, p 13). We feel that the illustrative case studies reflected the importance of carefully managing the creation, crafting, meaning and representation of boundary practices and objects, as well as the role of boundary spanners, in providing a high level of coherence in interprofessional practice.

References

Abbott, A. (1988) *The system of professions. An essay on the division of expert labor*, Chicago, IL: University of Chicago Press.

Arnkil, T.E. and Seikkula, J. (2015) 'Developing dialogicity in relational practices: reflecting on experience from open dialogues', *Australian and New Zealand Journal of Family Therapy*, 36(1): 142-54.

Barr, H., Koppel, I., Reeves, S., Hammick, M. and Freeth, D. (2005) *Effective interprofessional education. Argument, assumption and evidence*, Oxford: Blackwell.

Barton, J. and Parry-Jones, W. (2004) 'Adolescence'. in R. Detels, R. Beaglehole, M.A. Lansang and M. Gulliford (eds) *Oxford textbook of public health*, Oxford: Oxford University Press.

Bhaskar, R. and Danermark, B. (2006) 'Metatheory, Interdisciplinarity and Disability Research: a Critical Realist Perspective', *Scandinavian Journal of Disability Research*, 8(4) 278-97.

Bihari Axelsson, S. and Axelsson, R. (2009) 'Altruisme i tverrprofesjonelt samarbeid og ledelse' [Altruism in inter-professional collaboration and leadership], in E. Willumsen (ed) *Tverrprofesjonelt samarbeid i praksis og utdanning* [Cross-professionally cooperation in practice and education], Oslo: Universitetsforlaget, pp 104-15.

Callon, M. (1986) 'Some elements of a sociology of translation: domestication of the scallops and the fishermen of St Brieuc Bay', in J. Law (ed) *Power, action and belief: A new sociology of knowledge*, London: Routledge, pp 196-223.

Carlile (2004) 'Transferring, translating and transforming: an integrative framework for managing knowledge across boundaries', *Organization Science*, (1): 555-68.

Elvik, I. and Willumsen, E. (2011) 'Forbedringsarbeid og tvisteløsning i Stavanger' [Improvement work and dispute resolution in Stavanger], Article from the project 'Sammen for barn og unge' [Together for children and youth], Kommunenes Sentralforbund, available at www.ks.no/PageFiles/18606/Sammen_for_barn_og_unge_2.pdf.

Frenk, J., Chen, L., Bhutta, Z. A., Cohen, J., Crisp, N., Evans, T., Fineberg, H., Garcia, P., Ke, Y., Kelley, P., Kistnasamy, B., Meleis, A., Naylor, D., Pablos-Mendez, A., Reddy, S., Scrimshaw, S., Sepulveda, J., Serwadda, D. and Zurayk, H. (2010) 'Health professionals for a new century: transforming education to strengthen health systems in an interdependent world, *The Lancet*, 376(9756), 1923-1958.

Kjellevold, A. (2013) *Retten til individuell plan* [The right to an individual plan], Bergen: Fagbokforlaget.

Meads, G. and Ashcroft, J. (2005) *The case for interprofessional collaboration: In health and social care*, Oxford: Blackwell.

Molander, A. and Terum, L.I. (2008) 'Profesjonsstudier – en introduksjon' [Studies of professions – an introduction], in A. Molander and L.I. Terum (eds) *Profesjonsstudier* [Studies of professions], Oslo: Universitetsforlaget, pp 13-27.

Nonaka, I. (1994) 'A dynamic theory of organizational knowledge creation', *Organisational Science*, 5(1): 14-37.

NOU (Norwegian Green Paper) 2009:22 *Det du gjør, gjør det helt. Bedre samordning av tjenester for barn og unge* [What you do, do it completely. Better coordination of services for children and young people], Oslo: Barne- og likestillingsdepartementet.

Nowotny, H. (2003) 'Democratising expertise and socially robust knowledge', *Science and Public Policy*, 30(2): 151-6.

Oliver, C. (2013) 'Social workers as boundary spanners: reframing our professional identity for interprofessional practice', *Social Work Education*, 32 (6): 773-84.

Pawson, R. (2008) Reducing plague by drowning witches: Locating the real mechanisms of change in social and health interventions. Unpublished manuscript.

Payne, M. (2000) *Teamwork in multiprofessional care,* London: Macmillan.

Seaburn, D., Lorenz, A., Gunn, W., Gawinski, B. and Mauksch, L. (1996) *Models of collaboration*, New York, Basic Books.

Söderström, E. and Backman, A. (2011) 'Kraft genom samverkan – En abetsmodell för inledande samarbete' [Power through collaboration–a working model for initial cooperation], FSKC rapporter 4/2011, available at www.fskc.fi/Site/Data/2067/Files/PR_04_2011_FSKC%20Rapporter%204_2011d669(1).pdf.

Star, S.I. and Griesemer, J.R (1989) 'Institutional ecology, "translations" and boundary objects: amateurs and professionals in Berkeley's Museum of Vertebrate Zoology', *Social Studies of Science*, 19(3): 387-420.

Strauss, A. (1993) *Continual permutation of action*, New York, NY: Aldine de Gruyter.

Wenger, E. (1998) *Communities of practice: Learning, meaning, and identity*, Cambridge: Cambridge University Press.

Wheatley, M. J. (2007) *Finding our way: Leadership for an uncertain time*, San Francisco: Berrett-Koehler Publishers.

WHO (World Health Organization) (2010) 'Framework for action on interprofessional education and collaborative practice', available at www.who.int/hrh/resources/framework_action/en (accessed 7 August 2014).

Willumsen, E. (ed) (2009) *Tverrprofesjonelt samarbeid i praksis og utdanning* [Cross-professional cooperation in practice and education], Oslo: Universitetsforlaget.

Worrall, A. (2010) 'Boundary object theory', Paper presented at the LIS 6278 Seminar on Theory Development, Spring.

NINE

The formation of a profession: the case of physiotherapy in Norway

Eline Thornquist and Hildur Kalman

Introduction

Tasks and professions change over time, and theorists of professions such as Abbott (1988) emphasise that the development of a profession always takes place both through interaction and in conflict with adjacent professions. The tasks and fields of responsibility of a profession are the result of negotiations, struggles and border disputes with other professions. In the case of healthcare providers, the needs of different client groups and the state's wish for control and management are also part of the picture. In order to understand the development of a profession, it must be studied within an interacting *system* of professions. Task control – *jurisdiction*, according to Abbott – is in this connection the key to understanding.

In this chapter, we discuss the history of physiotherapy in Norway, which is a case that illustrates the significance of Abbott's perspective. It is first and foremost characterised by disputes related to the division of work and responsibility between physicians and physiotherapists, that is, jurisdictional borders concerning physiotherapists' practice and knowledge base. These disputes are closely connected to the struggle for acceptance by society, primarily expressed in the physiotherapist group's efforts to become part of the country's health services and to achieve public authorisation. A central concern with regard to physiotherapists' practice and knowledge base has been to have the state – not the medical profession – take control of the education of physiotherapists.

From the very beginning, in the early 20th century, physiotherapists – working in private institutes and with home visits – depended on physicians' acceptance and goodwill for a secure livelihood. Moreover, for 70 years physicians owned and ran the education of physiotherapists. As time passed, and as physiotherapists struggled for permanent positions in what became the country's welfare project, physiotherapy gradually developed as part of the state apparatus. Thus, and as we will show, the state should be regarded as a partner in strengthening the autonomy of Norwegian physiotherapists. This is the case with respect to crucial formalities, via legislation, as well as therapists' freedom at the workplace, for example, to choose new and relevant tasks and to broaden their client base. As to their training, the education of physiotherapists has for several decades been organised by the state.

First we focus on how physiotherapists in Norway tried to get control over their own field of work by attempting to obtain a framework that secured opportunities for good professional practice. Of particular importance is their struggle for social and organisational control through public authorisation and incorporation into the health service. We offer some examples of how gender came into play in the physiotherapists' struggles and the structural changes that were achieved. As an education's content and duration is of vital importance to any professional group's status, function and role in the community, we also explain how some of the milestones in the education sector were reached.

Physiotherapy in Norway: from the beginning

In 1895 the Sygegymnasternes Forening (Physiotherapists' Association, or SF) was founded by Louise Lyche who had received her education as a physiotherapist in Sweden. In addition to her, the members of the board were a physiotherapist, a cavalry captain and a physician. The latter two were men.

The SF board suggested a public education connected to the physical education college of the period. In this way gymnastics for the healthy and physiotherapy for the sick would complement each other, as they did at the Kungliga Gymnastiska Centralinstitutet (Royal Central Institute of Gymnastics, or RCIG) in Sweden, where the physiotherapists had been trained. But in a manoeuver reminiscent of a coup, the physician on the SF board started a private education institute in physiotherapy together with a colleague: Christiania Orthopædiske Institut (Christiania Orthopaedic Institute, or COI).

The Faculty of Medicine at the University of Christiania (currently Oslo) was consulted, where most of the physicians were critical of the proposal for a public education and for giving physical education for the healthy ample space. Their views functioned, in other words, as a legitimation of the establishment of COI. It is worth noting that the name of the school did not refer to the actual field of the education, but to 'orthopaedics' – a *medical* specialty.

The legacy from Sweden

In the 19th century and at the beginning of the next, before orthopaedics became a surgical specialty, orthopaedists and physiotherapists were real competitors. Disputes between the two groups were particularly noticeable in Sweden where physiotherapy – movement therapy – had a strong position (Holme, 1996; Ottosson, 2005). Both groups used various aids to relieve, support and correct faults, injuries and diseases of the musculoskeletal system, but the physiotherapists had in addition an *active* approach in their therapeutic toolbox.

The first school for physiotherapists in Norway was established at a time when the relationship between orthopaedists and physiotherapists was tense, and this sheds light on the original choice of name. The fact that 'orthopaedics' stayed part of the name until 1967, when the state took over responsibility for the education, has to do with the hegemonic position that medicine got in the health services in the 20th century. In other words, it is no coincidence that 'orthopaedics' became part of the school's name from the very beginning, nor that it was retained for so long.

Swedish education of medical gymnasts and the Ling tradition

RCIG was the leading institution in Nordic gymnastics and body culture throughout the 19th century and until the First World War, with a physiotherapy education that was well regarded far beyond the limits of the Nordic region (Lindroth, 2004; Ottosson, 2005).

That the Swedish state was the originator and stood as guarantor provided status. At this time, there was a new interest in gymnastics and body culture in Europe, and the general school system was considered to be a key instrument in ensuring physical education for new generations (Slagstad, 2010).

Per Henrik Ling (1776-1839) – known as the father of 'medical' gymnastics – headed RCIG from 1813 until his death. In his time, physiotherapy was an autonomous field with recognition and influence, and RCIG was an institution with little control from the outside. Ling was influenced by the new cultural trends from the continent, which emphasised the character-forming effects of gymnastics. He developed a system of movement characterised by discipline and *Bildung*, that is of moral and cultural cultivation. In Ling's posthumous (1840) work *Gymnastikens allmänna grunder* (*The general foundations of gymnastics*), health is presented as balance, disease as imbalance, and therapy as a way of mobilising nature's healing powers.

In accordance with their autonomy at this point in time, physiotherapists examined patients and developed individualised treatment programmes (Ottosson, 2005, p 78 onwards). With a double qualification as both physiotherapists and physical educators, the students of RCIG obtained the prestigious title 'director of gymnastics' after three years' education.

After Ling's death in 1839, RCIG's influence and good reputation continued, but eventually a series of reorganisations, driven by physicians with the aim of limiting the physiotherapists' room for manoeuver, began. In 1934, a decisive step was taken: gymnastics for the healthy and gymnastics for the sick were separated, and education in physiotherapy was moved from RCIG, reduced to one-and-a-half years and made subject to medical control. Physiotherapists lost the title of director, and their role was more or less to be assistants for physicians (Ottosson, 2011, pp 108-9).

The dramatic change in the status and autonomy of physiotherapists should be seen in the context of the emergence of bacteriology and a growing critique of natural philosophy during the last part of the 19th century (Shryock, 1979; Bynum, 1994). Throughout the 20th century, medical knowledge enjoyed increasing social acceptance in all western countries, and since the medical profession in Sweden gradually had been connected institutionally to RCIG, it created the premise for a development whereby physiotherapy was presented as its associated discipline.

Sweden differs from most other countries. In general, physiotherapists were historically the subordinates of physicians. Swedish physiotherapists started with a close connection to gymnastics and with a focus on health-promoting work; the first physiotherapists in other countries tended to work in hospitals where passive forms of treatment had a more central place (see, for example Barclay, 1994; Murphy 1995). Norwegian physiotherapy can be placed in an intermediate position. It started with one leg in medicine and the other in Swedish physiotherapy, and was placed under medical sovereignty under which gymnastics and movement therapy did not have the same elevated status as in Sweden.

Healthcare I: struggle for livelihood and public authorisation

For the first physiotherapists in Norway, the job market was difficult. They mainly worked in private institutes and with home visits (Haugen,

1997). Public positions in connection with social security offices around the country were created in 1914, and in hospitals in 1936.

With regard to the financing of practice outside hospitals, a reimbursement scheme was introduced in 1909 with the first law on medical insurance. In the later sickness benefit law of 1930, the patient got a social insurance right, which meant that social insurance was obliged to reimburse expenses for treatment by a physiotherapist. The condition for the reimbursement was that treatment was requested by a physician and performed by a physiotherapist with 'the required education'. With 'the required education', the emphasis was on whether or not the practitioner was 'authorised by a physician', a point to which we will return (Thornquist, 2014, p 153).

Working conditions deteriorated in the first decades of the 20th century. Physiotherapy was not well known, and it was difficult for therapists to support themselves. Massage was a popular form of treatment, and many others ran a massage business without any form of education, often as prostitution under the guise of massage. The physiotherapists wanted to make clear that they represented a decent profession. In this situation, they sought support from physicians, public authorities and women's organisations (Haugen, 1997, pp 98-110). Similar struggles took place in other countries as well (Nicholls and Cheek, 2006).

The Norwegian Medical Association created a Massage Council (Massageråd) that from 1918 gave a kind of authorisation to physiotherapists. Lacking legal significance, it still contributed to setting up professional barriers to disreputable competitors at the same time as physicians reinforced their position vis-à-vis physiotherapists.

It is worth noting that the Medical Association in the same year created a specialist scheme with 13 specialities, one of which was 'massage, medical gymnastics and orthopaedic treatment' (Haave, 2011). Thus, the physicians had secured their power base through two different institutional arrangements. In the decades that followed, physiotherapists engaged themselves strongly in the work to get public and legally binding authorisation, and a milestone was passed when public authorisation was achieved with the first law on physiotherapists in 1936 (Thornquist, 2014, p 147). Public authorisations function as jurisdictional seals of approval, and it was important for the physiotherapists to get both a protected enterprise and a protected title.

In 1936, another important event also took place, as a national association for Norwegian physiotherapists was established. In the decades that followed permanent positions in various parts of the health services were on the agenda, and rates in private practice was a recurrent theme.

Healthcare II: marking of the social mandate and physiotherapists' own competence

The Norwegian welfare state developed primarily in the post-war period, with particular growth and expansion in the 1970s (Seip, 1994; Hatlestad et al, 2006). The ties between the state and the professions are tight in Norway, as in Scandinavia in general. Throughout the 1970s, the government of Norway, like in other western countries, presented plans intending to reorganise the health services with greater emphasis on primary healthcare. The profession was strongly engaged in the effort to be incorporated into the welfare state projects.

The National Association of Physiotherapists, Norske Fysioterapeuters Forbund (NFF), argued that a better geographical distribution of physiotherapists was needed, and emphasised that private institutes rarely served children, the elderly and persons with severe functional problems. These demands created tension within the professional group; physiotherapists had a long tradition of being self-employed and running their own institutes, deciding themselves what categories of patients they wished to take on. Many physiotherapists simply did not want interference in their private enterprises. However, as NFF's views were in accordance with the aims and plans of the national authorities, they were met with approval.

A key point of the law was that each municipality now had the responsibility to coordinate the population's needs for different types of health services. This included the right to regulate private enterprises to some degree.

When the law on municipal healthcare was implemented in 1984, physiotherapy became a mandatory service in all municipalities. This meant that physiotherapists had increased their jurisdictional territory. Local authorities organised new, public positions with a fixed salary and established contracts with many, but not all, private practitioners.

With the municipal reform, physiotherapy was formally recognised as an important expertise in health services – an indication that the profession had achieved legitimacy. At the same time, the reform contributed to giving legitimacy (Kjølsrød and Thornquist, 2004).

However, as mentioned, there were physiotherapists who never endorsed NFF's views with regard to the municipal reform and a group of self-employed practitioners formed their own organisation, Privatpraktiserende Fysioterapeuters Forening (Association of

Physiotherapists in Private Practice, or PFF). PFF constitutes a clear minority of physiotherapists, its membership ranging between 400 and 900 since its foundation, surging to well over a thousand during the 2000s; there are at present approximately 14,000 authorised physiotherapists in Norway.

Healthcare III: referral scheme – control of tasks

A core issue in jurisdictional disputes vis-à-vis physicians has been the system of referral. Throughout the years, the system demonstrated a mismatch between physicians' formal power and ascribed role on the one hand, and their competence in physiotherapy on the other. The scheme had its formal basis in the physiotherapy law, section 7, stating that physiotherapists should not administer treatment 'without referral from a physician' (Thornquist, 2014, p 153).

The requirements for physicians' referrals to physiotherapists had varied over the years, and in 1971 they were sharpened: now physicians were obliged to state both the chosen treatment, and the duration and frequency of treatment for an insured person. Laws and regulations relating to self-employed practitioners had for a long time been a bone of contention, but now high on the NFF's agenda was the campaign to change the regulations so that they would be consistent with the physiotherapists' expertise and practice.

Physiotherapists found it unreasonable that they were not even allowed to adapt treatment to the individual patient with respect to time, measures and activities along the way. Also, it was essentially their own functional assessments – not medical diagnoses – that were the starting point for the selection of therapeutic approach.

In their daily work, physiotherapists in private practice always had considerable professional latitude; they have taken their decisions more or less independently of physicians' referrals. This was considered to be necessary because the referrals in general were unspecified and incomplete. All physiotherapists are familiar with the 'treatment package' that was frequently requested for many years: heat/massage/exercises – mostly expressed in abbreviated form 'h.m. + ex.'. Such standard formulations illustrate very clearly that thorough functional assessments of the individual patient did not form the basis of the physicians' referrals (see also Kjølsrød and Thornquist, 2004). The mismatch between formalities and reality was well known in both medical and physiotherapist circles, but both parties continued their practice in tacit mutual understanding, and cooperation – or the lack of it – between them created a few problems. It was in the formal jurisdictional area that the profession now made an effort to bring about change.

At the NFF's National Executive Committee meeting in 1985, physiotherapists' responsibilities and independence in the health services as a whole was on the agenda. Once again changes in the referral scheme were emphasised. The association was successful in some of its demands as a separate rate for examination was introduced that year, which meant recognition of physiotherapist assessment skills. The next step for greater autonomy was taken when the legal regulations were changed so that physicians in their referrals were 'allowed' to leave the choice of treatment to physiotherapists. This happened only in 1996 after several rounds of negotiations.

The developments in the case of referrals demonstrate that control over responsibilities was not something the Medical Association was going to give up voluntarily. A number of physicians had throughout many years 'given' physiotherapists a free hand in actual practice, but most physicians, and their association, nevertheless wanted to keep formal control. The fact that it concerned status-giving tasks such as examinations and treatment was presumably of some importance, given the hierarchy of tasks in health services. Another factor was that the physiotherapists' group was growing and kept making its mark more clearly.

Throughout the 1990s, the physiotherapists presented more radical demands. One concerned direct access – the right to examine and treat without a referral from a physician at all. When the physiotherapy law was abrogated and a new law on health personnel was implemented in 2001, the referral arrangement was cast in a new light. The formal basis for the referral scheme was removed, but the arrangement did not cease. From 2001, physiotherapists could indeed treat patients without a referral, but the state still chose to keep the profession under medical control as social security reimbursement was only to be given when there was a physician's referral – which is also the case today.

Gender and power

Let us have a closer look at two examples where gender has influenced historical transformations of physiotherapy, first by taking a retrospective look at Sweden in the 19th century, then by focusing on the municipal health reform in Norway in the 1980s.

Sweden in the 19th century

To begin with, education at RCIG was available only to men; women were admitted in 1864. So all physiotherapists in the period 1813 to 1866 were men (Ottosson, 2011, p 89). Half a century later, women were in the majority. How did this happen?

The changes in education mentioned already, which limited the room for manoeuver of physiotherapists, were promoted by physicians and entailed a 'de-masculinisation' of the physiotherapy profession (Ottosson, 2011, pp 106-8). Physicians had in 1929 even tried to stop men from getting access to the education of physiotherapy. Even if the attempt did not succeed, after the reorganisations at RCIG in 1934, the education was not as attractive for men as previously.

Ottosson emphasises that the physicians' strategies for de-masculinisation were directed against the autonomy of physiotherapists, not against physiotherapy as a field of knowledge (Ottosson, 2005, p 49). For the medical profession, it was important to obtain definitional power over everything having to do with health and illness, and this presupposed opposition to the male (autonomous and well-regarded) physiotherapists; it was a fight between men. As a consequence, the 'natural' gender hierarchy was established with men in roles superior to women's, which Ottosson calls a 'regendering of the physiotherapy profession' (Ottosson, 2005, p 386). 'The impulse ... is therefore not patriarchal structures which ... marginalise women', he writes, and continues: 'the fuel feeding the process of changes was the opposite, i.e. men's need to subordinate other men' (Ottosson, 2005, p 32).

Norway in 1980s

The struggle between physiotherapists over the municipal reform in the 1980s shows that the question of gender in professions is a complex and ambiguous phenomenon, which involves more than respective numbers of women and men. In physiotherapy, men and women represent different professional orientations and there is a clear division of gender in the labour market. After the reform, this was pushed to extremes. Positions with a fixed salary in the municipalities were, with few exceptions, occupied by women, while men continued to work in – and own – private institutes.

In other words, the reform reinforced the traditional division of work among women and men; in public physiotherapy services, women have always been in a majority, whereas most male physiotherapists work in private institutes. In the following decades, the gendered division of labour continued (Dahle, 1990; Enger, 2001). Male physiotherapists' interest in sports, training and manual therapy has continued, whereas women slowly have moved into the traditional male areas in line with the general development of society.

The educational sector I: the road to a public education run by the state

After the Second World War, there were continuous attempts to make the physiotherapy school a public institution. The students criticised the management (read: the physicians), requesting that the school keep up with professional developments and reflect society's need for physiotherapists.

In the 1950s and 1960s, several public committees were appointed, all of which gave futile recommendations that the state take charge of the privately owned school, until a committee was appointed with the mandate of making a plan for the establishment of a state school for physiotherapists. No longer an issue of public or private, the question now was what *sort* of state school it was to be, and when the plans could be implemented.

The committee's proposal conveys an instructive ambiguity concerning professional borders. On the one hand, physiotherapy was presented as an activity subordinate to medicine, and physiotherapy as a vocation controlled by physicians (for instance, physiotherapists were referred to as 'physicians' assistants'). On the other hand, it was repeatedly made clear that physiotherapists in actual practice had considerable autonomy.

The committee further suggested a one-year mandatory internship, and that training should be geared more to hospital and preventive work. These suggestions were all followed, and in 1967 the state took over the education of physiotherapists. Governmental running and a name showing the school to be a subject in its own right – Statens Fysioterapiskole, Oslo (State School of Physiotherapy, or SFO) – was the result of long-running attempts by the physiotherapists themselves, combined with an increasing political will to discontinue private educations. The next step was taken when the first physiotherapist – a woman – was hired as a headmaster at the school in 1974.

The educational sector II: professional borders, further education, academisation

To have the state as guarantor and regulator of physiotherapy practice and education did not mean that the need for marking professional autonomy was over. Border disputes with physicians were no longer the central issue, as state control entered the picture in ambiguous ways. Since the 1970s the educational field has been characterised by two tension-filled relations: on the one hand the relationship between an academic and practical/clinical tradition of knowledge, and on the other hand the relation between interdisciplinarity and professional borders.

A few years after the physiotherapists had acquired a state school, it was time for a new struggle – to keep the school an independent and unitary education institution. The authorities suggested a common and coordinated gradual educational model for several professional groups. After several years of massive opposition from the affected groups, parliament passed a resolution that there should still be separate educations for each professional group, suggesting they should be placed at the university college level (Thornquist, 2014, p 166). But the suggestions from the 1970s reappeared repeatedly over the following decades.

During the 1980s, most public documents on health and education suggested more emphasis on cooperation and interdisciplinarity. Now professional neutrality was the order of the day, and it was often stressed that the educational sector had a special responsibility for promoting a common sense of identity among health personnel (Thornquist, 2014, p 173).

The academisation process that had been going on in the physiotherapy profession for some decades was reinforced during the 2000s, especially by the reform of 2003, where all higher education was adapted to the division between the Bachelor, Master and PhD levels. After the turn of the millennium, Master's courses became the profession's academic alternative to further training arrangements that formerly had been run under the supervision of the union. Five Master's courses – all clinically oriented – were started during a period of five years. Given the tension between an academic and a practical tradition of knowledge, it is worth noting both the profile of these Master's courses and the considerable interest in them. It is clear that Norwegian physiotherapists were intent on continuing and developing the profession's practice traditions and that the desire was to combine the academic and practical/clinical competence.

Research in physiotherapy has grown rapidly. The field is characterised by a certain breadth, and by the year of 2016 about 150 physiotherapists had presented a doctoral thesis in Norway.

Conclusion and general remarks

Around the turn of the millennium, the Norwegian government emphasised the importance of health-promoting and preventative work, and physical activity and training were increasingly pointed out as important means of the healthcare sector. This was popular in physiotherapy circles; many physiotherapists now felt they were on home ground. With this, the wheel has turned full circle to the Ling tradition's emphasis on the health gain of movement and physical activity, even though the contents and knowledge base of physiotherapy has changed considerably, and as other groups of the population now benefit from physiotherapy.

Offering an account of the most important milestones in the history of physiotherapy in Norway, we have tried to demonstrate the importance of having a historical overview in the study of a profession, where transformations in areas such as the jurisdiction of professional practice and knowledge, organisation and economy are taken into consideration.

Decisive steps in the professional struggles of Norwegian physiotherapists have been taken both in the educational sector and in the health services. In both fields, the relationship between private and public organisation has been the fulcrum. Here it also becomes apparent how gender has been not only a question of the numbers of women and men in the profession, but how the processes of change have been gendered.

The health sector and society at large have undergone vast transformations in recent decades, encompassing processes that have not only expanded the territory of physiotherapists, but also changed professional relations on all levels. New institutional arrangements have brought new areas of work and new constellations among healthcare providers. Norwegian physiotherapists have achieved great independence compared with the first physiotherapists at the beginning of the last century. Today, physiotherapy is a profession in the health services in its own right, and collaboration with physicians is largely conflict-free.

We have strived to demonstrate how formal control – jurisdiction – is key in understanding the history of Norwegian physiotherapy, which supports Abbott's general point. In this book, several authors problematise control, referred to as New Public Management (NPM), where the authorities try to regulate and control professional practice. In line with these authors, we want to underscore the changing role of the state and how the audit culture of NPM (see also Powell,

1997) may come to clash with the professional aims and interests of physiotherapists.

A relatively common view of governmental control is expressed by two Australian physiotherapists when they write: 'Throughout its history, physiotherapy has been controlled first by medicine and more recently, by the state' (Kell and Owen 2008, p 160), and the authors express concern for a development where physiotherapists must 'act as *servants* of the state' (p 159, emphasis added).

However, as we have attempted to show, the majority of Norwegian physiotherapists have not regarded state control as something negative per se. This points to the importance of taking different dimensions of control into account, for a closer look at the effects of differing attempts for control of a profession, and for the professional practice in question.

External control in the form of the referral system and the physicians' control over education and work content has curtailed Norwegian physiotherapists' function and role, while control in the shape of authorisation and legislation connected to the health services has had more ambiguous effects. The authorities' emphasis on interdisciplinarity has to a certain extent limited physiotherapists' scope for action and employment of their expertise, but it has also had beneficial effects by securing the coordination of patients' treatment progress.

Physiotherapists have worked to protect and take care of their own competence, among other things through efforts to change the framework for the professional practice in terms of legislation, education and the organisation of health services. The profession has thus not only attached importance to good working conditions for itself, but has also been concerned with physiotherapy becoming available to groups that easily fall outside the private services. Thus, it can be said that the external control has served governmental principles of a just distribution of health services *at the same time* as it has served the profession's own interests.

However, in Norway – as in other welfare states – there are ongoing discussions about the organisation of welfare services, buzzwords being competition, outsourcing and privatisation.

The ties between the state and the professions are loosening in Norway, as in Scandinavia in general, as privatisation is steadily growing and is partly politically stimulated. An increasing interest for private enterprise is evident among Norwegian physiotherapists, a development fuelled by the contemporary concern with the body and health, producing a market for exercise and training. These changes are putting the tensions between the market versus the state, between interest in profitmaking versus social mandate, on the professional-political agenda anew.

References

Abbott, AD. (1988) *The system of professions. An essay on the division of expert labor*, Chicago, IL: University of Chicago Press.

Barclay, J. (1994) *In good hands: The history of the Chartered Society of Physiotherapy 1894-1994*, Oxford: Butterworth Heinemann.

Bynum, W.F. (1994) *Science and the practice of medicine in the nineteenth century*, Cambridge: Cambridge University Press.

Dahle, R. (1990) *Arbeidsdeling – makt – identitet: betydningen av kjønn i fysioterapiyrket* [Division of labour – power – identity: The importance of gender in the profession of physiotherapy], Trondheim: Institutt for sosialt arbeid, Universitetet i Trondheim.

Enger, K.J. (2001) 'Kjønn og spesialisering i fysioterapi' [Gender and specialisation in physiotherapy], *Fysioterapeuten*, 68(11): 16-22.

Hatlestad A., Kuhnle S. and Romøren TI. (eds) (2006) *Den norske velferdsstaten* [The Norwegian welfare state], Oslo: Gyldendal Akademiske.

Haugen, K.H. (1997) *En utdanning i bevegelse: 100 år med fysioterapiutdanning i Norge* [An education on the move: 100 years of education in physiotherapy in Norway], Oslo: Universitetsforlaget.

Holme, L. (1996) *Konsten att göra barn raka. Ortopedi och vanförevård i Sverige till 1920* [The art of making children straight. Orthopaedics and care for the disabled in Sweden until 1920], Stockholm: Carlssons Förlag.

Kell, C. and Owen, G. (2008) 'Physiotherapy as a profession: where are we now?', *International Journal of Therapy and Rehabilitation*, 15(4): 158-64.

Kjølsrød, L. and Thornquist, E. (2004) 'From a liberal occupation to an occupation of the welfare state. Norwegian physiotherapy 1960-2000', *Acta Sociologica*, 47(3): 277-89.

Lindroth, J. (2004) *Ling – från storhet till upplösning: Studier i svensk gymnastikhistoria 1800-1950* [Ling – from greatness to dissolution: Studies in Swedish history of gymnastics 1800-1950], Eslöv: Brutus Östlings bokförlag Symposion.

Ling, P.H. (1840) *Gymnastikens allmänna grunder* [The general foundations of gymnastics], Uppsala: Leffler och Sebell.

Murphy, W.B. (1995) *Healing the generations: A history of physical therapy and the American Physical Therapy Association*, Lyme, CT: Greenwich Publishing Group.

Nicholls, D. and Cheek, J. (2006) 'Physiotherapy and the shadow of prostitution', *Social Science & Medicine*, 62(9): 2236-48.
Ottosson, A. (2005) *Sjukgymnasten – vart tog han vägen? En undersökning av sjukgymnastyrkets maskulinisering och avmaskulinisering 1813-1934* [The physiotherapist – where did he go? A study of the masculinisation and de-masculinisation of the physiotherapy profession 1813-1934], Göteborg: Historiska Institutionen, Göteborg Universitet.
Ottosson, A. (2011) 'The manipulated history of manipulations of spines and joints?', *Medicine Studies*, 3(2): 83-116.
Power, M. (1997) *The audit society*, Oxford: Oxford University Press.
Seip, A.L. (1994) *Veiene til velferdsstaten* [The ways to the welfare state], Oslo: Gyldendal Forlag.
Shryock, R.H. (1979) *The development of modern medicine*, Madison, WI: University of Wisconsin Press.
Slagstad, R. (2010) *(Sporten): en idéhistorisk studie* [(The sporting section): A study related to the history of ideas], Oslo: Pax Forlag.
Thornquist, E. (2014) 'Fysioterapeutene. Fra kosmologi til fagpolitikk' [The physiotherapists. From cosmology to trade union politics], in R. Slagstad and J. Messel (eds) *Profesjonshistorier*, Oslo: Pax Forlag, pp 138-76.

TEN

The professional development of social work in Poland after 1989

Sabina Pawlas-Czyz, Lars Evertsson and Marek Perlinski

Introduction

In modern European welfare states, professionals like nurses, physicians and social workers have a prominent role as they provide social and medical care and services to citizens. However, their practice is not always for the good of the client. They may also serve as gatekeepers in the sense that they restrict citizens' access to welfare services, and it is their mandate to monitor, educate and discipline citizens' moral conduct (Titmuss, 1968; Bertilsson, 1990).

A close connection to the welfare state has been favourable, and for some professions even decisive, for professional development. Previous research on welfare professions shows that the welfare state plays a central role in creating new jurisdictions, or bringing change to already established jurisdictions. Through its political commitment to social and medical services, the welfare state engages and shapes the welfare professional landscape by demarcating professional jurisdictions, allocating resources to education and research and certifying professional credentials that regulate the licence to practise (Evertsson, 2000; Wrede, 2001; Evertsson and Lindqvist, 2005). But the welfare state is not always an ally. It can push professions in a direction they do not want to go, or even marginalise or extinguish them (Evertsson, 2002). In this chapter we give an example of the latter, that is, how the welfare state has acted against the interest of the social work profession. The example comes from Poland where the jurisdiction of the social work profession has taken a direction that is not in line with professionals' aspirations.

Our main contribution in this chapter is to show how the jurisdiction of welfare professions such as social work is sensitive to changes in welfare policy. More precisely, we argue that welfare policies are a structuring link between the state and the professional jurisdiction.

Theoretical points of departure

In research on professions, the concept of jurisdiction is frequently used to describe the knowledge and practice fields that a profession claims to control (Abbott, 1998). For welfare professions, jurisdictional control is closely related to, and conditioned by, the welfare state. Professional jurisdiction is intimately woven into the fabric of politics since it is tied to services and resources set by the state. Unlike market-based professions, it is almost impossible for professions that operate within the realm of the welfare state to claim jurisdiction or offer services that are not in line with existing social policies. Their dependency on the state therefore makes them sensitive to changes in welfare policy. Research shows that in order to protect or develop their jurisdiction, welfare professions need to act in the political arena, that is, to influence or pressure the state to design policy in a way that serves the professional group in question. To reform the professional landscape by political actions can be seen as a strategy of politicisation (Åmark, 1990; Torstendahl, 1990).

The development of the social work in Poland: social and political background

Social work as professional practice and profession hardly existed in Poland before 1989 when Poland became a democratic republic. Prior to 1989, social services had a marginal position. They was run and controlled by the Ministry of Health and Social Care (Ministerstwo Zdrowia i Opieki Społecznej), targeting social emergencies and covering basic social needs. The weak legislative framework, and lack of staff and organisational resources, meant that most citizens had no access to social services. The meagre resources that did exist were primarily used to support citizens who through disability or sickness were permanently unable to work.

To understand the marginal position of social work in Poland, it is necessary to go back to the so-called Stalin period (1948-56). During this period it was officially declared that social work was not needed since the state denied the existence of social problems. The Stalin period effectively put a stop to pre-war efforts to establish social work as professional work in Poland. Most of the legislative Acts on social work from 1923 were cancelled, schools giving professional training within the field of social work were forced to close, institutions providing social care were shut down, and the responsibility of social care was transferred from local authorities to the state. However, at the beginning of the 1960s, attempts were made to reintroduce social work. Parts of the pre-war social care Act were re-enacted, some institutions providing social care was reopened and, building on its pre-war roots, schools providing training within the field of social work started to re-emerge (Wódz, 1996).

However, the state of social work in the late 1980s was not up to meeting the challenges that emerged when Poland broke with its socialist past. Social problems that were previously denied came to fore and the shift to a market economy created new social problems. The lack of trained social workers, legislative framework and local authorities within the field of social work made social services both ineffective and insufficient.

Against this background a new Social Care Act (Ustawa o pomocy społecznej) was enacted by parliament in 1990. The new Act changed the marginalised position of social work in Poland. The act gave social work and social workers a prominent position within the provision of social services and opened up a new jurisdiction for social work as a profession.

The Ministry of Labour and Social Policy (Ministerstwu Pracy i Polityki Społecznej) was commissioned to design the new landscape of social services and to arbitrate over the division of responsibilities between the state and local authorities. It also established the professional qualifications required to practise social work and delineated the tasks and services that would fall under the jurisdiction of social work. The Ministry of Labour and Social Policy concluded that social workers main tasks fall within two different areas of social services: preventive care and activation and independence. Preventive care included services providing material and economical support, while activation and independence included services with the intent to support 'individuals and families in strengthening or regaining the ability to function in society' (Ustawa o pomocy społecznej z dnia 29 listopada 1990 roku, article 8).

In conjunction with the Social Care Act, the education of social workers gained political interest. There was a shortage of trained social workers that needed to be addressed, and the content of social work education had to be brought in line with the new jurisdiction. As a result, several universities were granted permission to start education in social work at both Bachelor and Master's level.

The revival of the social work profession in Poland

Seen from an analytical perspective, it is reasonable to argue that the introduction of the Social Care Act in 1990 signifies the birth of social work as a modern profession, social work as professional practice and social work as a university subject and research field.

However, social workers were only able to take possession in half of the intended areas of jurisdiction. The state and the local authorities focused their resources on preventive social work at the expense of services aiming at supporting individuals and families in strengthening or regaining the ability to function in society. Put another way, the original idea that social workers should run two kinds of parallel programmes – one with a focus on preventive care, and the other with a focus on activating clients and making them independent – were not realised in practice. Therefore, the jurisdiction that was opened up for social workers came to focus on preventive social work, mainly providing material and economical support.

The political focus on prevention should be seen in the light of the profound transformation of Polish society that followed the process of democratisation and the introduction of a market economy. The system changes left many people in dire straits and financial poverty (Rymsza, 2012). However, the lack of services targeting clients with more complex social needs was not only a matter of priority, but also reflected a flux in the socio-political infrastructure on which the Social Care Act rested. Put another way, the long-standing tradition that social services were run and controlled by the state was not easily replaced, and local authorities struggled to find administrative forms for their new responsibilities within social services.

The focus on prevention gave social work an administrative character. Social workers' main task was to perform needs assessment and their main professional role to exercise public authority and make a formal decision on who was eligible to material and economic support. Within the educational system, however, social workers were still trained for their original jurisdiction, which included work with dysfunctional families and clients with complex social needs.

Jurisdictional losses and gains: the introduction of the family assistants

Gradually, a new socio-political landscape came into being, and in the early 2000s the postponed plans to provide social services to dysfunctional families and clients with complex social needs gathered new momentum. To target the social needs of these groups, two new social political reforms were introduced in 2010 and 2011. In 2010 the Social Act on Preventing Family Violence was introduced (Ustawa o przeciwdziałaniu przemocy w rodzinie) and in 2011 the Social Act on Family Support and Foster Care (Ustawa o wspieraniu rodziny i systemie pieczy zastępczej).

Seen from the perspective of the social work profession, the new reforms were a disappointment. In both Acts, social workers were given a marginalised position. In fact, the services aimed to meet the needs of dysfunctional families and clients with complex social needs were not defined as social work in these Acts. In the Social Act on Preventing Family Violence, social workers were given an administrative role, for instance assessing the need for and making the decision about whether or not to place children in social care.

The social work profession was given the same administrative role in the Social Act on Family Support and Foster Care. The tasks of providing support to improve the life situations of families, solving social and psychological problems, giving advice on questions relating to children's upbringing, training and supporting parents' parental skills, motivating family members to increase their professional qualifications, and helping in the search for work were given to a new profession – the family assistant. The profession of family assistant was open to anyone with a university degree in sociology, psychology or pedagogy. Those with university degrees in other subjects, but with a qualification in child and family work, could also enter the profession. Social workers were also qualified to gain access to the new profession, on the condition of giving up their professional status as social workers.

The rationale behind the reform and the introduction of the new profession was to strengthen professional work with children and families with complex needs. The Social Act on Family Support and Foster Care marks a shift in Polish social policy since it focuses on the family, and views social problems as a mismatch between resources and capacities within families and demands in society. The previous system of social services was criticised as being insufficient since it targeted the individual rather than the family. It was argued that existing social services were not organised and lacked the capacity to work with the family as a system.

The need of system-based changes to improve social services for children and families with complex needs was postulated a number of times (Racław, 2012). In its ambition to improve professional work with children and families with complex needs, the government made an organisational split between social workers and the new profession, family assistants. The government concluded that the existing model of organisation of child and family care did not support the intended direction of change.[1] As a result, professional work within the Social Act on Family Support and Foster Care was placed outside of the organisation and jurisdiction of the social work profession. From a theoretical point of view, it is reasonable to suggest that the organisational demarcation between social workers and family assistants in combination with well-defined tasks and clients created a distinct jurisdiction for the family assistants.

But why did the state choose to create a new profession and jurisdiction instead of using experienced and well-educated social work professionals? On this issue the records are not all clear. However, nothing indicates that the marginalisation of the social work profession was a reflection of critique against the profession. A more plausible motive seems to have been the limited number of social workers. To expand the jurisdiction of the social work profession to include children and families with complex needs would have had negative consequences on their work since social workers were the only profession trained to perform needs assessments and qualified to exercise public authority within the area of material and economic support. Hence, their marginalised position were more likely a reflection of their specific professional competence in combination with the limited number of social workers available, that is, the numbers of social workers were insufficient to inhabit the new services targeting children and families with complex needs within a reasonable time. Put another way, the marginalisation of social workers was a matter of their specific professional competence and labour supply rather than a disqualification of their competence to work with children and families. Seen from the perspective of the state, recruiting family assistants from those with a university degree in sociology, psychology, pedagogy – or those with a degree in another subject, but with additional training in child and family work – made it possible to establish a profession within a relatively short time.

The university departments of social work and the social work profession were critical of the introduction of a new jurisdiction within the field of social services. They argued that the social work profession was trained and qualified to provide the services that were specified within the Social Act on Family Support and Foster Care. It was also pointed out that the social work profession had worked with children and families with complex social needs in municipalities prior to the Social Act on Family Support and Foster Care and experimentally introduced family assistantship as a modern form of social work within municipalities. As a method of supporting children and families with complex needs, family assistantship was first introduced in the Social Care Centre of Sopot (Rudnik, 2010). Several models were developed, and in most cases the professional role of family assistant was performed by a social worker (Kowalczyk, 2012). As Trawkowska (2007) noted, social workers were professionally prepared for working with children and families and had a good knowledge of local issues. Therefore, to build on their expertise would further the professionalisation of services aimed at children and families with complex needs.

Given these circumstances, the university departments in social work and the social work profession argued that these services should fall into the jurisdiction of social work, but they did not win the ear of the state. However, as mentioned earlier, the social work profession was not totally excluded in the Social Act on Family Support and Foster Care: the administrative role that was assigned to social workers placed them in a position where they gained control over diagnosing and assessing the needs of families with care and educational difficulties. Social workers were also given the role of supporting and assisting family assistants in planning social interventions.

The social Acts from 2010 and 2011 consolidated the bureaucratic and administrative role of the social work profession. However, at the same time, they represent an expansion of social work jurisdiction since they put social workers in the position of supporting and managing the work of family assistants.

Deprofessionalisation versus professionalisation of social work

The situation in Poland raises questions concerning whether these developments represent a deprofessionalisation of the social work profession or an increased professionalisation. One answer to that is that it depends on what we choose to focus. Some may argue that the social work profession in Poland is going through a process of deprofessionalisation since there is a discrepancy between their jurisdiction and professionals' own vision of social work and what ought to belong in their jurisdiction. Arguments of deprofessionalisation are fuelled by comparing social work in Poland with that in other welfare states.

However, it is also possible to argue that the social workers in Poland have strengthened their professional position within the broad field of social services. The Social Acts from 2010 and 2011 can be seen as an expansion of their jurisdiction since it gave social workers a bureaucratic and administrative role where they support and control the professional practice that is carried out in accordance with these Acts. This development can be seen as an expression of a continued professionalisation of the social work profession. Seen from a theoretical point of view, it is reasonable to argue that the social work profession in Poland aimed at obtaining full jurisdiction (Abbott, 1988) within the broad area of social services, that is, complete, legally established control over what social workers consider to be the heartland of social work. They lost that battle but that does not mean they are on the slope of deprofessionalisation. The notion of an ongoing deprofessionalisation of social work in Poland might be nothing more than a reflection of what the profession regards as professionally desirable and prestigious rather than actual deprofessionalisation. Given the social work profession's position, it is possible to argue that there is a divided jurisdiction (Abbott, 1988) between social workers and family assistants within the Social Act on Family Support and Foster Care. The social worker's main task is to perform needs assessment and exercise public authority, that is to make formal decisions regarding who is eligible to social services, whereas the family assistant's task is to work directly with children and families and their problems. Put another way, within the policy field of family support and foster care, social workers function as case managers – making assessments and allocating resources – while family assistants are responsible for the hands-on work with children and families – so-called micro-practice (Kaźmierczak, 2012). The notion of a divided jurisdiction is supported by the peaceful co-existence between social workers and family assistants. Family assistants view social workers as one of their most important partners in their work to support children and families while social workers view family assistants as important allies in their work (Pawlas-Czyż, 2014).

However, as professional jurisdiction is shaped by, and tied to, welfare policies this peaceful co-existence might change in the future. There are also signs indicating that the social work profession has not giving up its aspiration of incorporating direct client work with children and families within its jurisdiction. In many municipalities social workers try to develop and improve methods for working with children and families with complex needs in order to change the division of professional work between the professions (Kowalczyk, 2015). This kind of professional action might change the peaceful jurisdictional truce of today that rests on a functional division of professional labour.

Conclusion

In this chapter we have argued that welfare policies can be seen as a structuring link between the state and the professional jurisdiction, and that welfare professions because of that are sensitive to changes in welfare policies. We have showed how the jurisdiction of the social work profession and family assistants has been shaped by the welfare political ambition of the Polish state within the broad field of social services.

Based on previous research, we also argued that welfare professions, in order to protect or develop their jurisdiction, need to act in the political arena, that is, to influence the policymaking process by the strategy of politicisation. However, in the case of the social work professions in Poland, it seems that this strategy has been of limited use. It is seems that the social work profession and the university departments of social work have lacked the bargaining strength to influence the state to grant them a jurisdiction that encompasses direct client work with children and families with complex social needs, which the profession opted for. Our empirical data therefore suggest that the social work profession and the university departments of social work have not succeeded in using the strategy of politicisation in this case. One way to understand the lack of bargaining strength could be that it takes time to build political networks and alliances, and to muster the organisational resources necessary to successfully negotiate with the state. The modern social work profession in Poland only goes back to the early 1990s.

The lack of bargaining capacity may shed light on why the social work profession has not managed to position itself as a welfare professional solution within the policy field of family support and foster care. However, seen from the perspective of the state, developing social services within this new field of family support and foster care was not only a matter of proper professional skills, but also a question of how to recruit and staff this new field of social services quickly, especially how to find enough manpower. To this question the social work profession was not a viable solution in the eyes of the Polish state. Given their long professional training, it would take considerable time to staff the area of family support and foster care with social workers. There were not enough trained social workers to fill the positions within the new emerging area of social services. Transferring social workers from their position within social services would not have solved the shortage, but would only have resulted in shuffling the problem from one area to another, since no other professionals were trained to perform needs assessments or qualified to exercise public authority within the area of material and economic support. It is reasonable to assume that the shortage played an important role in the state's search of a professional alterative to social workers, and in the decision to create the profession of family assistant.

The Polish case illustrates that professional development that takes place in close partnership with the welfare state is in no way an easy process to control for the professions. It also illustrates that professionalisation that occurs within the realm of the welfare state is more than a mere reflection of professional competence; it is a political process where professional competence is set against other factors, for instance labour supply and staffing issues. Seen from a theoretical point of view, this is interesting since much of the literature on the sociology of the professions tend to emphasise the role of education, credentials and scientifically based knowledge in studying and understanding professional development. The core idea is that professional knowledge is a resource that can be used in the labour market and exchanged for money and social prestige (Parkin, 1979). Hence, to strengthen professional status and position, it is vital to develop and protect the knowledge base. This strategy often includes an element of controlling the size of the profession, for example limiting the supply of professional labour on the market to make sure it does not exceed demand.

This perspective might serve as a good starting point when studying market-based professions. However, when professionalisation occurs within the welfare state and takes the shape of politics – rather than following the logic of the market – there might be other scarce resources that are as important as knowledge (Evertsson, 2002). Drawing on the Polish case, it looks like one of the reasons that the social work profession got 'bumped' in favour of an entirely new profession was that labour supply was deemed a more scarce resource than professional competence in relation to the social services that was going to be implemented. Events in Poland point to the limitations of building a professional strategy solely based on knowledge. Social workers were professionally qualified, but their exclusive character – few practitioners with a long and specialised university training – became a constraint in the situation where the state did not primarily look for the best available competence, but for a large number of practitioners who were good enough.

The Polish case can also serve as a starting point to reflect on interprofessional conflicts and competition. Within the sociology of the professions there is a tendency to view inter-professional competition as a central driving force for making jurisdictional claims and setting jurisdictional disputes. However, given the situation in Poland where social workers and family assistants have overlapping jurisdictional claim, which does not seem possible to resolve through competition or conflicts, cooperation might be a better strategy. To cooperate could increase social workers' bargaining strength vis-à-vis the state and facilitate the use of politicisation. For cooperation to occur both professions must have something to gain. For the social work profession there are obvious gains to be had. For many social workers the concept of social work is particularly important for their understanding of professional identity (Niesporek et al, 2013). Cooperation with family assistants might be their best chance to get access to direct client work and to bring their work and identity more in line with what they consider to constitute the core of professional social work. Seen from the perspective of social workers, gaining access to direct client work is vital to developing their professional practice and profession role. As shown in this book and by others, direct client work is of utmost importance for social workers' understanding of professional identity (Perlinski, 2010). Research shows that Polish social workers experience a problem of double identity, caused by the tension between their current position within social services and the lack of a direct client relationship, considered to be the core of social work (Bieńko, 2012). The key question, however, is what does the family assistant gain by cooperation?

Note

[1] The government project justification of the Act on Family Support and Foster Care, Warsaw 16 September 2010, print no 3378, 128-161; orka.sejm.gov.pl.

References

Abbott, A. (1998) *The system of professions. An essay on the division of expert labor*, Chicago, IL: University of Chicago Press.

Åmark, K. (1990) 'Open cartels and social closures: professional strategies in Sweden, 1860–1950', in M. Burrage, and R. Torstendahl (eds) *Professions in theory and history,* London: Sage Publications.

Bertilsson, M. (1990) 'The welfare state, the professions and citizens', in R. Torstendahl and M. Burrage (eds) *The formations of professions. Knowledge, state and strategy*, London: Sage Publications.

Bieńko, M. (2012) 'Dylematy profesji i roli w refleksyjnym projekcie tożsamości współczesnego pracownika socjalnego na przykładzie pracowników powiatowych centrów pomocy rodzinie' [Dilemmas of the profession and the professional role in a reflective project about identity of contemporary social worker in county family assistance centers], in M. Rymsza (ed) *Pracownicy socjalni i praca socjalna w Polsce. Między służbą społeczną a urzędem* [Social workers and social work in Poland. Between social service and administration], Warszawa: Instytut Spraw Publicznych, pp 93-120.

Evertsson, L. (2000) 'The Swedish welfare state and the emergence of female welfare state occupations', *Gender, Work and Organization*, 7(4): 230-41.

Evertsson, L. (2002) *Välfärdspolitik och kvinnoyrken. Organisation, välfärdsstat och professionaliseringens villkor* [Welfare politics and female dominated occupations. Organization, welfare state and the conditions for professionalization], Umeå: Umeå Universitet, Sociologiska Institutionen.

Evertsson, L. and Lindqvist, R. (2005) 'Welfare state and women's work – the professional projects of nurses and occupational therapists in Sweden', *Nursing Inquiry*, 12(4): 256-68.

Kaźmierczak, T. (2012) 'Pracownicy socjalni, kapitał ludzki, profesjonalna praktyka' [Social workers, human capital, professional practice], in M. Rymsza (ed) *Pracownicy socjalni i praca socjalna w Polsce. Między służbą społeczną a urzędem* [Social workers and social work in Poland. Between social service and administration], Warszawa: Instytut Spraw Publicznych, pp 159-86.

Kowalczyk, B. (2012) 'Modele pracy asystenta rodziny i współpracy z pracownikiem socjalnym' [Work models for family assistants and their cooperation with social workers], *Praca Socjalna*, 4: 3-15.

Kowalczyk, B. (2015) 'Asystent rodziny, pracownik socjalny – jeden zawód? Refleksje na marginesie standardów pracy socjalnej z rodziną' [Family assistant, social worker – one profession? Reflections on the margin of standards of social work with family], in B. Chrostowska, M. Dymowska and M. Zmysłowska (eds) *Rodzina wobec problemów i wyzwań współczesności. W poszukiwaniu rozwiązań* [Family and the problems and challenges of the present. In the search of solutions], Olsztyn: UWM.

Niesporek, A., Trembaczowski, Ł.and Warczok, T. (2013) *Granice symboliczne. Studium praktyk kulturowych na przykładzie działań zawodowych pracowników socjalnych* [Symbolic boundaries. Study of cultural practices on the example of professional activities of social workers], Kraków: Nomos.

Parkin, F. (1979) *Marxism and class theory. A bourgeois critique*, London: Tavistock Publications.

Pawlas- Czyż, S. (2014) 'Koordynator pieczy zastępczej we współpracy z asystentem rodziny a formuła case management' [Coordinator of foster care in cooperation with the assistant. The case management formula], *Trzeci Sektor*, Special volume, 2013/14: 91-105.

Perlinski, M. (2010) *Skilda världar – specialisering eller integration i socialtjänstens individ- och familjeomsorg* [Separate worlds – specialization or integration in the personal social services], Umeå: Umeå Universitet, Institutionen för Socialt Arbete.

Racław M. (2012) 'Zmiany w pracy socjalnej z rodziną – w stronę kontroli stylu życia i zarządzania marginalizacją' [Changes in social work with families – towards control of lifestyles and management of marginalization], in M. Rymsza (ed) *Pracownicy socjalni i praca socjalna w Polsce. Między służbą społeczną a urzędem* [Social workers and social work in Poland. Between social service and administration], Warszawa: Instytut Spraw Publicznych, pp 227-44.

Rudnik, M. (2010) 'Asystentura rodzin realizowana w ośrodkach pomocy społecznej w Polsce' [Assistantship for families in social assistance centers in Poland], in M. Szpunar (ed) *Asystentura – nowa metoda w pomocy społecznej w Polsce* [Assistantship – a new method of social assistance in Poland], Gdynia: MOPS, pp 31-47.

Rymsza, M. (2012) (ed) *Pracownicy socjalni i praca socjalna w Polsce. Między służbą społeczną a urzędem* [Social workers and social work in Poland. Between social service and administration], Warszawa: Instytut Spraw Publicznych.

Titmuss, R.M. (1968) *Commitment to welfare*, London: Allen & Unwin.

Torstendahl, R. (1990) 'Essential properties, strategic aims and historical development: three approaches to theories of professionalism', in M. Burrage, and R. Torstendahl (eds) *Professions in theory and history. Rethinking the study of the professions*, London: Sage Publications.

Trawkowska D. (2007) 'Niewidoczna czy nieistniejąca. Praca socjalna z rodziną w pomocy społecznej' [The invisible or non-existent. Social work with the family in social assistance], in B. Matyjas and J. Biała (eds) *Rodzina jako* środowisko *pracy socjalnej. Teoria i praktyka* [Family as social work setting. Theory and practice], Kielce: Wydawnictwo Akademii Świętokrzyskiej.

Wódz, K. (1996). *Praca socjalna w* środowisku *zamieszkania* [Social work in client's place of residence] (2nd edn), Katowice: Wydawnictwo Śląsk.

Wrede, S. (2001) *Decentering care for mothers. The politics of midwifery and the design of Finnish maternity services*, Åbo: Åbo Akademi University Press.

ELEVEN

Professional dilemmas of defining a problem: the case of addiction treatment

Joakim Isaksson and Daniel Törnqvist[1]

Introduction

Let us start this chapter with a question: if you had a drug problem, to which profession would you go to seek help? If we think about this question for a couple of seconds, it seems naive, almost provocative in its simplicity. If we live in a welfare state, this is one of the things we should know, and if we do not, we should be able to find out without much effort. However, we do think that this question has to be raised in order to problematise other basic sociological questions, namely: where does the drug problem belong? Which profession is best suited to help people with drug problems?

As we all know, how we as a society view and define a problem is not self-evident, and depends on a number of factors. As a starting point, we can use some of the thoughts formulated by Berger and Luckmann (1966), namely that:

- Reality is something we construct together through social interaction.
- What we see as knowledge is an object for the sociology of knowledge.
- Different professions are defined and 'guarded' by different mechanisms where knowledge plays a crucial part.

To expand on the latter point, and in the words of Berger and Luckman (1966, p 105):

> Meanwhile the fully accredited inhabitants of the medical world are kept from 'quackery' ... not only by the powerful external controls available to the profession, but by a whole

> body of professional knowledge that offers them 'scientific proof' of the folly and even wickedness of such deviance. In other words, an entire legitimating machinery is at work so that laymen will remain laymen, and doctors doctors....

This example concerns physicians, and serves well as an introduction to this chapter, in which we discuss two different professions, namely 'physicians', as representatives of medical science, and 'social workers' as representatives of social sciences. Addiction and addiction treatment is an interesting case since physicians work together with other professions in a way that is not evident in other areas. For instance, we have a hard time imagining a patient with a broken bone going to social services, or someone who has just been evicted as being primarily in need of a doctor's appointment. That is not to say that there are not a number of professional groups working with and helping individuals with drug problems (psychologists, drug counsellors and so on), but the focus in this chapter will be limited to these two professions since the debate about drug problems in Sweden has mainly been related to these two professions in terms of treatment.

Aim of the chapter

Using Sweden as an example, our aim is to analyse and discuss how the use of drugs has been defined at different time periods and how these different definitions may cause dilemmas for the welfare professions involved in addiction treatment.

In order to analyse and problematise these questions, we will give examples of how the use of (narcotic) drugs has been discussed in Sweden. Although the empirical examples clearly are bound to the Swedish social context, we do believe that the analysis and reasoning put forward is valid in other contexts as well. In the following, we offer a brief historical overview of different perspectives on drugs and drug use and how addiction treatment is organised in Sweden. Thereafter, we present three empirical examples in order to show how changes in policy and perspectives have taken place in the 2000s. This development is analysed in the light of medicalisation. Finally, we conclude the chapter by pointing out some professional dilemmas associated with defining a problem based on different ontological assumptions.

Historical perspectives on drugs and drug users in Sweden

The use of drugs was recognised as a serious societal problem in Sweden around the mid-1960s. Surely, narcotics were used earlier than that, but by groups that were not perceived as a threat to society in the same way as young people using, for example, amphetamines and cannabis as part of a sub-culture (Lindgren, 1993; Olsson, 1994).

In the 1970s, drug use was, by and large, perceived as something *new*, which also meant that there was no consensus on how to look at drug use, for example in terms of what caused it, how it should be treated and so on. Furthermore, during this period and up to the 1990s, the dominant view was that drug use was a *social* problem, and therefore should be treated with social interventions.[2] A number of examples can be given to support this claim. Social workers and those working in the treatment of drug users were very active in the debate, and supported the 'social view'. The explanations for drug use were, for example, a harsh and competitive society, stress and inhumanity, and the unjust organisation of society and its resources. So, in a way the debate over drugs during the 1970s and 1980s can be seen as a form of *social criticism*. Similar opinions were also expressed by many of the politicians active in the debate (Törnqvist, 2009). A good illustration of this from the 1980s comes from Gertrud Sigurdsen, a member of the Swedish parliament:

> The group now appointed by the government represents a large amount of knowledge about drug use: the National Board of Health and Welfare, the National Police Commissioner, the Correctional Treatment system, the Board of Customs etc. The fight against drugs is mainly a task for these authorities; with support from organisations such as Parents Against Drugs.... The fight against drugs is to a very little degree a medical problem. (Dagens Nyheter, 1989-11-11, authors' translation)

Furthermore, non-governmental organisations (NGOs) such as Parents Against Drugs (Föräldraföreningen mot narkotika) and the National Organisation for a Drug-Free Society (Riksförbundet för ett narkotikafritt samhälle) had a prominent role in the debate, and were strongly opposed to a drug policy including what we now would call harm reduction actions. Clearly, this illustrates how strong the support was for a social explanation of drug use, and how physicians and medical knowledge by and large was considered irrelevant in this field.

Although physicians were active in the debate during these 30 years, their contributions almost exclusively defended medical interventions (needle-exchange programmes and substitution treatment), which met with strong criticism from other debaters.

During the 1990s, however, Swedish drug policy became subject to criticism, mainly from the academic field, where a number of social science scholars argued that the current politics did not produce positive results, and had several negative side effects: labelling young people as criminals, a high death-rate among opiate users with severe problems, a high economic cost and so on (Törnqvist, 2009). In a way, this may be seen as a criticism of the hegemonic perspective on social explanations of drug use, which, in turn, opened up the field for new understandings of the problem and sufficient treatments.

Recent Swedish context

Before we show some empirical examples in order to support our claims, that is, that new understandings of the problem of drug use and drug users have arisen, we believe it is necessary to provide the reader with some basic facts about the organisation of Swedish welfare.

First, healthcare is organised in what is called regional healthcare authorities (*landsting*). They are the ones planning, organising and caring out healthcare. There are 20 regional healthcare authorities in Sweden.

Second, social services (among many other things) are organised and carried out by one of the 290 municipalities in Sweden. Both municipalities and regional healthcare authorities (as well as the Swedish parliament) are run by a political assembly chosen every four years.

It is important to know this because care given by the Social Services Act, including addiction treatment, compulsory treatment of addicts and compulsory treatment of young people, is the responsibility of the municipality. In everyday life this may not seem to matter very much, and of course the organisations work together (since they often try to help the same people). A person could, for example, come to the emergency room because of an overdose, and when that person is stable the social services might be involved, and the client may end up at a treatment facility. However, it seems reasonable to interpret the placement of addiction treatment under the remit of the municipalities as an important statement that drug use was primarily seen as a social problem.

However, during the 2000s, some changes in policy have been carried out, and a slightly different view on drugs and drug users has surfaced.

Even if Sweden still has a strict policy when it comes to narcotics – not only possession but also consumption is criminalised – there are some indicators that we might be heading towards a slightly different approach to drugs and drug users. We now turn to three examples that point towards such a new approach.

Needle-exchange programmes

Programmes for needle exchange are a common form of help available to intravenous drug users in many countries. It became increasingly popular as a form of intervention with the discovery of the HIV virus in the 1980s. Traditionally, this approach had been very restrictive in Sweden, and had strong opponents in the NGOs. The arguments given to support this position were, for example, that the programmes did not work properly (people with addiction problems did not bother to access them) and that drug users continued to share the new needles. Furthermore, the programmes were thought to be sending mixed messages by providing known drug users with injection needles even though drug use had been criminalised since 1988 (not just possession as had been the case previously). This had the effect of placing the care provider in the legally 'grey' zone of actually helping someone to commit a crime. Nevertheless, in 1975, permission was given for the cities of Lund and Malmö to establish strictly supervised needle-exchange programmes.

In the middle of the 2000s, the minister of public health Morgan Johansson changed the policy so that every regional healthcare authority could decide whether they wanted to offer drug users this form of treatment. The change in policy did not come with any proclamation that the formerly repressive Swedish politics had been proven ineffective, but was presented merely as an opening for more people with drug problems to get access to this form of treatment. To summarise, an intervention that previously came under heavy criticism was suddenly deemed by policymakers to be rather unproblematic. Furthermore, it was treatment *within the healthcare system* that was the focus.

Substitution treatment

The use of opioids[3] as a form of treatment for opiate addicts had had a history of nearly 50 years at the time of writing.[4] It is a form of treatment aimed not at achieving a drug-free life, but a life without withdrawal symptoms. The theory is that this, in turn, should help individuals to take care of other parts of their life: a place to live, employment and so on.

Much like the situation with needle-exchange programmes, the attitude in Sweden towards this form of care was originally very restrictive. Nevertheless, the first programme of this kind in Europe was started in Ulleråker in Sweden as early as 1966. It was strictly supervised, had a maximum number of patients, and stood for a minimal part of the total addiction care in Sweden. In the 1980s and 1990s, three more clinics opened up in Stockholm, Lund and Malmö.

The current situation is yet another one altogether. Since buprenorphine was introduced as a complement to methadone (one advantage being that it is less toxic), and then Subuxone, which besides buprenorphine contains the opiate antidote Naloxon, the number of patients in substitution treatment has skyrocketed in Sweden. Certainly there are guidelines and regulations governing the programmes for substitution treatment, which are overseen, handled and revised by the National Board of Health and Welfare (Socialstyrelsen). Since the first programme started, there have been several different versions, but the changes have pointed in one direction: it has become easier to get access to this form of treatment. It is also an outspoken goal that the treatment should be offered to a larger number of clients. Although it is difficult to explain the entire changes solely with the introduction of new pharmacological products (factors such as drug users' awareness of the treatment, cultural and social changes and so on may also be considered), it is still interesting to take a look at some numbers in this area.

- Treatment is now provided at over 100 clinics in Sweden.
- From 2005 to 2011, the number of clients increased by 600%, from approximately 860 to 5200 (National Board of Health and Welfare, 2012).

Obviously, numbers like these illustrate the following fact clearly: substitution treatment has become a significantly bigger part of addiction treatment in Sweden than before. And again, it is mainly within the medical field that these changes have taken place.

A commission for better treatment

Our third and final empirical example concerns a public investigation ordered by the government in 2011 with the title 'Better interventions for addiction and dependence' (SOU, 2011:35). The investigation concerned the situation regarding substance abuse, current research and so on, and came up with a number of suggestions in order to improve addiction treatment in Sweden. What is of most interest here was some of the suggestions that were put forward. One of them was that the regional healthcare authorities and *not* the municipalities should be responsible for addiction treatment. The overall responsibility would therefore shift from social services to the medical field and the medical professions. Another suggestion was that medication should become a bigger part of addiction treatment, not only for substitution treatment, but also for clients with alcohol problems. In short, medication was not considered to be used enough. When it came to substitution treatment, one suggestion was that people addicted not only to opiates, but to opioids as well, could be considered for treatment. Other suggestions together give the picture that substitution treatment is a form of care that more clients should be able to access.

This example goes hand in hand with the earlier two, and again, it is within the medical field that answers are sought; it is medical interventions that are the focus. Although the investigating commission did not deny the importance of social and psycho-social interventions as part of the treatment as well, the overall trend towards a new (medical) understanding of drugs and drug users was clear.

Medicalisation

The empirical examples might easily be understood in the light of medicalisation,[5] which has been of interest to sociologists for the past 40 years (Zola, 1975; Freidson, 1988; Conrad and Schneider, 1992; Conrad, 2005). This concept refers to a process by which non-medical problems become defined and treated as medical problems, which, in turn, mandates or gives license to the medical profession to provide some type of treatment for it (Zola, 1975; Conrad, 1992). The process of medicalisation is, however, a broad definitional process and occurs on at least three distinct levels; the conceptual, the institutional, and the interactional level (Conrad, 1992). On the conceptual level, a medical vocabulary is used to define the problem at hand, usually through medical labelling. The institutional level refers to how organisations adopt a medical definition and approach to a problem, although non-medical personnel accomplish the everyday work. Finally, on the interactional level, physicians are more directly involved as part of the doctor–patient interaction by defining a problem as medical and treating a social problem with a medical form of treatment (Conrad, 1992).

One important aspect of medicalisation is that it involves processes of different types of social control depending on how a problem is understood. To further the understanding of this, Conrad and Schneider (1992) developed a theory of the 'bright' and 'dark' side of understanding a problem in medical terms. Issues related to the bright side of such a process relates to the positive and empowering effects that a medical definition might have for the individual. Most prominent of these are increased tolerance and compassion, the removal of blame and the portrayal of an optimistic outcome. By and large, all these issues are related to a more humanitarian social control in medicine that is easier for the individual to handle. However, in contrast, the negative individual outcomes are related to the masking of the social. This means that a medical understanding of a problem is supposed to mask social factors as the cause of the problem, that is, the individual is seen as the problem bearer and attention is diverted from the organisational as well as the political level. Due to this, the main criticism of such processes is that it tends to decontextualise and individualise what might otherwise be interpreted as collective social problems (Conrad, 1992). Hence, by expanding medical interpretations and jurisdictions of a problem to new arenas, there is a great risk that the impact of organisational and societal conditions are obscured.

Taking the empirical examples mentioned earlier into consideration, it seems reasonable to claim that a medicalisation of drug use has escalated during latter years in Sweden on several levels. For example, in order to receive substitution treatment, an individual has to be categorised or diagnosed as a drug addict by a physician (conceptual level), that is, individuals have to portray themselves as being biologically or medically deviant (as opposed to having a complicated life situation). Furthermore, although substitution treatment rarely involves a typical patient–physician relationship, the physician still holds a prominent place in the system by defining the problem as medical and prescribing treatment, for example in terms of buprenorphine or methadone. Finally, and perhaps most important, this process is most visible on the institutional level considering the fact that treatment in clinics has increased drastically during the 2000s, but also that policymakers increasingly advocate medical prescriptions to a wider group of addicts, for example opioid addicts. Furthermore, the suggestion of transferring the responsibility of addiction treatment from the municipality to the regional healthcare authorities also supports these claims.

Different perspectives, different professional dilemmas

So far, we have shown how the problem of drug use has been defined in Sweden at different times, and have interpreted this development in terms of a process towards a medicalisation of drug use in recent years. To summarise this discussion, Table 11.1 provides a brief overview of the two perspectives and how they differ on a number of levels, which in turn have consequences for the treatment provided. It also shows the scientific origins of each definition and its ontological assumptions.

Since tables often become a bit dichotomous, it should merely be thought of as an illustration of ideal types, that is, mental constructs (Weber, 1949). Hence, the difference between the perspectives is not that clear-cut in reality. However, professions with different perspectives often aggressively claim jurisdiction over their area of expertise (and

Table 11.1: Summary of the two perspectives on drug problems

	Medical problem-definition	Social problem-definition
Ontology of drug problems	Drug problems refers to individual characteristics and a biological sensitivity towards drugs – individual focus.	Drug problems are caused by social circumstances – social criticism.
Disciplinary basis	Medicine/science	Social science
Implications for treatment	The individual body in focus. Medication/substitution treatment/medical interventions.	A situational focus. Social interventions with a broader scope. More focus on the life situation and social circumstances of the individual rather than individual characteristics.
Reasons for drug use and treatment	Biomedical causes. Substitution treatment is needed in order to reduce the symptoms of the individual's addiction.	Social circumstances of the individual, for example structural barriers in society and unequal distribution of welfare resources. A harsh and difficult life situation or personal crises might trigger drug use.
Function in the welfare state	Administrative function – a diagnosis/medical definition as a condition for taking part in substitution treatment.	Care-oriented definition guided by an ambition to understand the individual's addiction in a wider societal context. Less bound to resources and specific treatments – depends on the individual.

their perspective) and the members of that profession carry out its practices to the best of their abilities in line with their ontological assumptions about a problem. For a physician, this may be searching for certain things in blood tests, while for a social worker, it may be interviewing a client using the MI method.[6] *However, our main point is that when the different professions look for certain things and put certain things in the foreground, they necessarily put other things in the background.*

The mention of ontology earlier needs further elaboration, since it illustrates another dilemma relevant for this chapter. We have in this chapter discussed physicians – as representatives of the medical science – and social workers – as representatives of the social sciences. One should bear in mind that these two fields of science originate from very different backgrounds, and therefore rest on different ontological and epistemological assumptions. Medicine, with its roots in the positivist tradition, has a more materialistic view of the world, and from an epistemological stance, focuses more on empiricism – empirical experiments to see whether a hypothesis should be accepted or rejected.

Social sciences on the other hand, can be said to have a more idealistic view of the world, or, to borrow from Thomas Kuhn, they represent another paradigm (Kuhn, 1962) – a different belief system governing which scientific questions are deemed relevant, which methods should be used to answer them and so on.[7]

Given this, it is also a fact that medical definitions of problems (usually in terms of medical diagnoses) often are considered as more 'objective' than other explanations, which, in turn, makes physicians a strong group as 'gatekeepers' in the welfare state's fair distribution of resources to vulnerable groups. This may also be an explanation of why professions other than the medical profession use a medical perspective on certain (social) problems, especially if they experience less legitimacy for their own interpretations of the problems in the welfare system.

Well then, do these differences in the theory of science matter? To that, we would like to answer both no and yes. No in the sense that we do not believe that in the day-to-day work of addiction treatment – whether it is done by physicians, social workers or some other profession – ontological discrepancies are what are perceived as one of the major problems. But, if we want to understand why these discrepancies occur, and how it can be that we sometimes look at problems so differently, then absolutely yes.

Surely, it is desirable that both perspectives are used in line with a holistic approach and this is also the main idea in addiction treatment where physicians and social workers often work together. However, we must also keep in mind that professions often want to gain jurisdictional control over their work and clienteles and therefore compete with other professions in the same field (Abbot, 1988), including striving to 'hegemonise' their perspective on a certain problem. Hence, this may create certain dilemmas when trying to achieve multidisciplinary work where several perspectives should be used in order to decide on the best care for the client. Furthermore, the fact that one perspective or paradigm always becomes dominant makes this work even more problematic and might make other professions 'abandon' their own professional perspective.

This problem may be illustrated by turning to a completely different problem that has become subject to a process of medicalisation in Sweden in recent years, namely learning difficulties experienced by pupils in school. Quite similar to the environment of addiction treatment, schools encompass several different occupational groups representing different professions and academic disciplines. Investigations into whether a pupil might be considered to have special needs is performed by a multidisciplinary team, including the school nurse, the principal, a special educationalist and a social worker. The main idea behind such a multidisciplinary team is that the different professions should use their own perspective on the problem (social, medical or pedagogical) so that all perspectives are covered, that is, a kind of holistic approach. However, a great amount of research has shown that the medical perspective is dominant among most of these occupational groups – even the non-medical professions. For example, in a study of such teams, Hjörne (2004) found that staff used well-established institutional categories and seemed to systematically individualise pupils according to a biomedical model of explanation. Clearly, this shows that the dominance of one perspective might be very problematic in practice and might also weaken the other professions' own assumptions about the problem. Furthermore, strong support from policymakers for one perspective might also produce doubts among other professions and less legitimacy for their perspective.

Conclusion

This chapter shows how different definitions of a problem may cause dilemmas for professions involved in addiction treatment.

Using Sweden as an example, we have argued that there has been a tendency towards an increasing medicalisation of drug use during latter years, which, in turn, may cause certain dilemmas for the welfare professions involved in addiction treatment, dilemmas that we think are important to consider for both current and future practitioners in the welfare sector. One such dilemma concerns which professional group is best suited to be responsible for addiction treatment: social workers or physicians? The current situation, and one that will probably continue, is that they are both involved, but which profession has jurisdiction over the problem is not self-evident. However, as we have shown, one should keep in mind that these perspectives do have consequences for the treatment provided and for how reasons for drug use are interpreted (whether they are based on individual or contextual factors). Another dilemma concerns the fact that these two professions represent two schools of science, and although it may not seem like a big problem for current and future practitioners, it is our firm belief that it is worth reflecting on. What does the 'lifting' of a problem from one scientific discipline to another mean and what are the implications of this for the individual?

As teachers in a social work programme, we have witnessed how students take on a medical perspective very early during their studies. Although it is important to accept other professions' perspectives and points of departure, and to be open about different understandings of a problem, it is just as important to stand up for assumptions and knowledge of one's own profession. Otherwise, what's the point of collaborating with other professions?

Notes

1 The authors contributed equally to the preparation of this chapter, and are listed alphabetically.

2 This view did not necessarily change during the 1990s, but the discussion about what causes drug use did not get the same attention as before.

3 The term 'opioid' usually refers to drugs with opium-like effects (natural and synthetic), while 'opiates' are used to refer to analgesis derived from the opium poppy (natural). Thus, all opiates are opioids but only some opioids are opiates.

4 Traditionally methadone, but since the 2000s as buprenorphine (Subutex and Subuxone).

5 Some authors, however, now find the term 'biomedicalisation' more appropriate to use in order to capture how the expansion of medical power and knowledge have been displaced and changed due to biotechnological developments (Clarke et al, 2003). Whereas previously the driving forces of medicalisation often were associated with the medical profession and patient activism, the driving forces today are more likely to be associated with the pharmaceutical industry, the role of technoscience and patients'/consumers' increasing demands for pharmaceutical products.

6 Motivational interviewing: a certain approach/method used in counselling.

[7] The reasoning is extremely basic, but will hopefully illustrate our point. A lengthier discussion can be found in any textbook in the field of theory of science; see, for example, Potter (2000).

References

Abbott, A. (1988) *The system of professions. An essay on the division of expert labor*, Chicago, IL: University of Chicago Press.

Berger, P.L. and Luckmann, T. (1966) *The social construction of reality. A treatise in the sociology of knowledge*, New York, NY: Penguin Books.

Clarke, A.E., Shim, J.K., Mamo, J.R., Fosket, J.R. and Fishman, J.R. (2003) 'Biomedicalization: technoscientific transformations of health, illness, and US biomedicine', *American Sociological Review*, 68(2): 161-94.

Conrad, P. (1992) 'Medicalization and social control', *Annual Review of Sociology*, 18(1): 209-31.

Conrad, P. (2005) 'The shifting engines of medicalization', *Journal of Health and Social Behaviour*, 46(1): 3-14.

Conrad, P. and Schneider, J. W. (1992) *Deviance and medicalization: From badness to sickness*, Philadelphia, PA: Temple University Press.

Freidson, E. (1988) *Profession of medicine. A study of the sociology of applied knowledge*,Chicago, IL: University of Chicago Press.

Hjörne, E. (2004) *Excluding for inclusion. Negotiating school careers and identities in pupil welfare settings*, Gothenburg: University of Gothenburg.

Kuhn, T.S. (1962) *The structure of scientific revolutions* (3rd edn), Chicago, IL and London: University of Chicago Press.

Lindgren, S.-Å. (1993) *Den hotfulla njutningen: Att etablera drogbruk som samhällsproblem 1890-1970* [The threatening pleasure: Establishing drug use as a societal problem 1890-1930], Stockholm: Symposion Graduale.

National Board of Health and Welfare (2012) *Kartläggning av läkemedelsassisterad behandling vid opiatberoende* [Mapping of medication-assisted treatment for opiate dependence], Stockholm: National Board of Health and Welfare.

Olsson, B. (1994) *Narkotikaproblemets bakgrund – Användning av och uppfattningar om narkotika inom svensk medicin 1839-1965* [The background to the narcotic problem. Use and ideas about narcotics in Swedish medicine 1839-1965], Stockholm: CAN.

Potter, G. (2000) *The philosophy of social science: New perspectives*, Essex: Pearson Education.

SOU 2001:35 *Bättre insatser vid missbruk och beroende* [Better interventions for addiction and dependence], Stockholm: Department of Health and Social Affairs.

Törnqvist, D. (2009) *När man talar om knark – drogdebatt i svensk dagspress 1970-1999* [When talking about drugs – Drug debate in Swedish daily press 1970-1999], Umeå: Umeå University.

Weber, M. (1949) '"Objectivity" in social science and social policy', in E.A. Shils and H.A. Finch (eds) *The methodology of the social sciences*, New York, NY: Free Press.

Zola, I.K. (1975) 'Medicine as an institution of social control', in C. Cox and A. Mead (eds) *A sociology of medical practice*, London: Collier-Macmillan.

TWELVE

Challenges of municipal community work

Witold Mandrysz, Marek Perlinski and Lars Evertsson

Introduction

Community work, in different forms, is a relatively common feature of social work in several European countries, although the concept itself was developed in Great Britain (Popple, 1995; Twelvetrees, 2008). Community work and social development aims to take advantage of citizens' initiatives, preferences, abilities and often hidden and sometimes forgotten resources, in order to achieve social change improving the living conditions of groups of citizens. Usually, community work is not purely a spontaneous, bottom-up process; it is typically initiated by specific stakeholder and actors. Non-governmental organisations often initiate the process, while authorities and institutional actors remain in the background. In some cases, however, the authorities initiate community work.

The aim of this chapter is to show the problems that are associated with attempts to bring about community work in neighbourhoods subject to urban decay. Community work and social development in demoted areas are sometimes, at least partly, initiated by local authorities seeking cooperation with inhabitants. The chapter focuses especially on the difficulties professional social workers face in such situations. One major difficulty is caused by the multiple, often contradictory, roles and multiple loyalties of social workers.

The empirical base of this chapter is a case study conducted during a social development project in a disadvantaged urban area of a medium-sized Polish town. The degradation of the area is an effect of the transformation of the Polish society and economy after 1989 when the country left the socialist plan economy behind and started on the path of western-type economy. During the socialist era, state companies had a great part in delivering social welfare services, sometimes even including housing for the workers. All that changed after 1989, partly due to disappearance of many companies, and the duty of delivering social services was taken over by local administration and authorities. They were to large extent unprepared for this. The local authorities were not fully developed and were also forced to work with existing (and emerging) social legislation, which was rudimentary and under-developed.

Today social development projects in Poland are usually planned, initiated and implemented by institutions acting on behalf of local authorities that oversee and control the implementation of these projects. Thus, they are top-down actions, which the authorities can carry out using EU structural funds. A typical example of such a project is the Kaufhaus residential area in the city of Ruda Śląska, which is used as a case study in this chapter. A Kaufhaus can be described as a social housing area where the prevalence of social problems is high.

The Kaufhaus case shows very clearly how difficult it is for local authorities to implement social development projects. Although it was not a total failure it, was not a success either. It showed the outmost importance of good understanding of the needs and problems of inhabitants; precise determination of priorities of action and possibility of allocation of available resources, such as participatory budgets; efficient information for prospective participants to prevent surprise and negative reactions when the activities are initiated; quick feedback on emerging problems before they take unmanageable proportions disturbing social peace; an increase in citizens' trust in the authorities and support for future actions of local authorities.

The chapter begins with a short introduction of the public governance concept, followed by a discussion of community work and social development in the Polish context. Thereafter the Kaufhaus case is introduced, which is preceded by a presentation of the main stakeholders of the social development project in Kaufhaus. The main part of the chapter is concerned with social workers' and inhabitants' experience of the project. The chapter ends with a summarising and concluding section.

Public governance and community work

The concept New Public Management (NPM) was developed in the wake of criticism of modern welfare states, and promoted among other things privatisation of public services (McLaughlin et al, 2002). In Poland such privatisation gave some consumers of public services the right to choose service provider; other consumers, however, found that their access to public services became limited. A counter-reaction to

NPM resulted in the development of the concept 'public governance' in the context of public services, which, among other things, means that citizens are seen not only as clients, but also as co-producers. By promoting the inclusion of stakeholders and citizens in the process of producing services, this idea came very close to the idea of community work (Giza-Poleszczuk and Hausner, 2008). Public governance refers to the active inclusion of consumers and beneficiaries in the production of public services, which is supposed to lead to improved quality and an increased range of services. Hence, public governance in principle is a manifestation of civic participation in conducting public policy, as well as involvement in actions and projects for common good at the local level. Community members can ideally obtain additional benefits through their own empowerment, and along with it have influence over the scope and quality of services.

Insufficient public resources forces welfare states to seek solutions that on the one hand are directed to entire communities, not only to individuals, and on the other hand are based not only on the involvement of public authorities and institutions, but also on other social actors and the residents themselves. In practice, social work of this type is usually defined as local community organising or community work. Such a combination of social and institutional resources significantly increases the chances of success of such activities, but also exposes them to the risks associated with locus of control and conflicts of interest (Mayo, 1998, p 162).

Community work and social development in a Polish context

Local community organising is defined as action, usually professional, which aims to mobilise and support members of the community taking action together to improve their own situation and to promote social development (Ross, 1967; Cohen, 1978; Rothman and Tropman, 1987; Wódz, 1998; Wódz and Kowalczyk, 2014).

Community organising is a chain of logically related activities that come together in a problem-solving process. This problem-solving process includes: defining or uncovering the problem; building the structural and communicational links for action on a problem; laying out the alternative options; adopting a strategy or policy; developing a plan and implementing it; and receiving feedback, monitoring process, and redefining the problem (Ecklein and Lauffer, 1971; Cox et al, 1987; Rothman and Tropman, 1987; Haynes and Holmes, 1994).

Thus, local community organising is a form of 'self-organisation' of inhabitants of a given territory enhanced by actions taken by specialists, professional animators, coordinators or organisers whose task is to integrate members of a given community around a given project. This requires specific, interdisciplinary knowledge, skills and competences.

Community organising is a planned process, with specific objectives clearly defined from the outset of the project. It requires an efficient centre for the coordination of the management and decision making.

Diagnosis of the problems and needs of a given community should not be based on an administrative decision or a suggestion made by specialists in social planning. It should build on a genuine inventory of needs expressed by inhabitants within this community. Broad social consultation is crucial. Only then do the members of any given community become experts in building priorities and strategies of action, not mere consumers of the support programmes but also their co-authors. This often brings about the necessity to conduct mediation, by creating a dialogue between community representatives, local authorities and representatives of local business sector whose interests may collide. Unfortunately, in a situation where the organiser of the local community is a social worker employed by the welfare institutions, it is difficult to talk about the possibility of impartiality and independence. Local community organisers are, to a certain degree and more or less officially, forced to act primarily in the interests of the local authority. Thus, they are at risk of losing not only independence, but also the trust of the community.

In Poland, the initiators and implementers of local community organising projects are usually local government institutions, along with the subordinated social assistance services. This is mainly due to the necessity to mobilise considerable financial resources in the areas under the jurisdiction of local authorities.

Theoretically the phenomenon discussed in this chapter can be understood as social development (Payne, 2005, pp 217-23). In Weil's typology we can find a model of community social and economic development, which refers to a group of people making up a territorial whole, yet being characterised by a sort of social or economic discrimination. The undertaken actions encourage poor and marginalised communities to take social and economic initiatives, which constitute the basis of the economic development of these groups of people and at the same time lead to the improvement of the economic or social conditions of their inhabitants (Weil, 2005). In this kind of community work model, particular importance is given to understanding local conditions affecting social relations, and the relations between residents and the local authority and its activities. As stated by Mayo:

> Community workers need to have knowledge and understanding of the socio-economic and political backgrounds of the areas in which they are work, including knowledge and understanding of political structures, and a relevant organisations and resources in the statutory, voluntary and community sectors. And they need to have knowledge and understanding of equal opportunities policies and practice, so that they can apply these effectively in every aspect of their work. (Mayo, 1994, p 74)

The Kaufhaus case

Kaufhaus is a residential area in a city of Ruda Śląska in south-western Poland. The city has 142,000 inhabitants. This region of Poland is still characterised by its past as one of Europe's heavily industrialised areas of coal mining and steel production in the period from the late 1700s to early 2000s, resulting in a symbiosis between industry and community. Social services, housing and communications were built up to serve the labour that coal mines and smelters needed.

Kaufhaus was a patronage estate at Pokój smelter in Ruda Śląska, founded in the late 19th and early 20th century. Its extensive service infrastructure made it almost self-sufficient. The smelter was the main provider of both housing and other services, and even medical infrastructure, satisfying almost all of the residents' needs.

The 1980s and 1990s were a period of decline and restructuring of the industry in the region. The patronage housing estates were usually brought into the municipal housing stock. Kaufhaus was modern for the time when it was founded, but is currently out-dated and degraded, not meeting modern hygienic and functional standards. The area has become a low price variant of municipal social housing inhabited by people with multiple social problems.

There are still some inhabitants that remember Kaufhaus as it once was.[1] They talk about how cosy life was in the 'good old days'. They remember a sense of familiarity and interpersonal bonds. Familiarity meant mutual help and support, spending time together, mutual unannounced visits, joint holidays and participating in other events important for the community, even leaving the doors unlocked giving the neighbours unfettered entry to each other's flats.

> "Here, life was good, here the people helped each other, and everyone knew everyone. It was such a family, maybe it was due to the fact that then more or less everyone had equally and everyone had hard. The people more respected each other as I remember from my childhood. They even lent things to each other if there was something lacking. The doors were never closed." (A woman of 65, a resident of Kaufhaus)

Currently, about 680 of 1,300 households in the Kaufhaus depend on some form of assistance from the municipal social services (social welfare centre). The main social problems among inhabitants include poverty, unemployment and addictions. In several residents' opinion such an accumulation of social problems in one place causes lack of good role models that could counterbalance negative behaviour. The weakening – or disappearance – of social bonds has led to the lack of attachment to 'new inhabitants' in the Kaufhaus, and thus its degradation.

> "It deteriorated when the city took it over.... because it is treated like a ghetto. Here the worst element comes. In one place there is an accumulation of the poor, the ones who do not pay the rent, drunks, etc. And what I think – is probably not the case, it should not be like that. In one place a motley collection of people and pathologies." (A man of 66, a resident of Kaufhaus)

The accumulation of social problems, according to the respondents, causes a decline of social control in the area, and thus an accelerated process of 'pathologisation' in the rest of the population and the dissemination of negative patterns of behaviour. This creates a strong sense of injustice and harm among the residents, who consider the local government and the authorities to be responsible for the difficult situation. It also fuels conflict between old and new residents. The whole residential area became a problem area with an accumulation of social problems, which prompted local authorities to engage in community work to achieve social development.

Stakeholders of the project

A Local Activities Programme (LAP) for the Kaufhaus settlement has been in force since June 2008 when the city council of Ruda Śląska approved a resolution on its adoption. The programme is integrated with a systemic project, 'Ruda Śląska – a chance for all', implemented by the social welfare centre in Ruda Śląska, and financed by the European Social Fund.

The objective of the project is social and professional integration of the local community. The project targets economically disadvantaged social welfare clients. More specific objectives are to create conditions for the emergence of initiatives and structures beneficial for the local community, to mobilise people at risk of social exclusion by improving their professional skills, developing their ability to job search, raising social skills, increasing their motivation to change their lifestyle, and building and consolidating mechanisms of self-help. Other objectives were creating a space for civil dialogue,[2] changing the negative image of the Kaufhaus settlements and its inhabitants, and strengthening inhabitants' engagement in the local community.

The programme, in the first year of its implementation, covered about 50 people at risk of social exclusion and their families. These individuals signed agreements concerning their rights and obligations as beneficiaries of the programme. These agreements, however, did not take the form of social contract. In 2009, the number of new participants was reduced to 30 people. In 2010 only 20 contracts were signed, mostly due to reduction of funds allocated to the project.

The main tools for solving social problems, and achieving social activation of people at risk of social exclusion, included socially useful assigned work, and courses in social and professional skills, communication skills, professional training and so on. Socially useful assigned work involved participants who were unemployed without the right to unemployment benefits.

Activities for the organisation of the local community comprised educational and cultural meetings, mainly art classes for children and adults, music lessons and photographic activities. These activities were directed to all residents of the Kaufhaus on the basis of voluntary attendance, although they were compulsory for people who had signed agreements on participation in the LAP.

Social workers' and residents' experience of the project

Although the LAP for Kaufhaus in Ruda Śląska[3] was implemented by the social welfare centre, it relied, at least to start with, on social workers who had not worked as social workers in the area. At that time, the organiser's cooperation with the local community was very good, according to organisers as well as residents. In a later phase, organisers were either social workers who previously had worked in the area, or were employed as social workers in the community. The later phase of the project meant that the social workers had dual roles. They were both the driving force (animators) and the municipal employees (official persons representing the local authorities). These dual roles created a number of difficulties.

Social workers with dual roles were not fond of such duality:

> "... it does not work at all, because 'the beneficiaries of the programme' and the other of the settlers did not want to take part in cultural and educational programmes implemented by these animators/social workers. This was due to the perception of a social worker by the residents – an official/clerk who requires, controls, who provides benefits, but can also withdraw them, a person with whom you should be careful what you say, so not to reveal additional, non-registered sources of income, etc." (Social worker working in Kaufhaus district)

Moreover, resident might feel that they were monitored and controlled by social workers and that decisions were made over their heads.

The final stage of the project created a new difficulty. At this stage the animators were people recruited by the local authorities from outside of the municipal welfare centre. The new personnel worked with a very limited number of active participants, about a dozen. The resources and possibilities of action were also cut down. The actions were restricted to cultural and educational activities at the headquarters of the LAP.

Residents of the Kaufhaus displayed poor knowledge of the project and also of what the municipality had actually done to improve the residential area. The residents were demonstrably unaware of infrastructure investments the municipality had made. This lack of knowledge was one important reason for their dissatisfaction with the project.

There are two reasons that may explain residents' lack of knowledge about the project. The first is a general trend towards individualisation of life, and a lack of willingness to engage in activities in the neighbourhood and community, in combination with weakened social bonds. The second reason may be a lack of adequate methods to engage citizens in the process of project implementation. Hanging posters, handing out leaflets and making announcements at open meetings are not effective enough. Such methods are especially ineffective in environments with a particular degree of social exclusion, where residents are predominantly reluctant to engage with local authorities. In such cases it is crucial to actively involve the inhabitants in the planning of activities. Planning together disseminates the goals and objectives of such projects and helps with understanding the planned activities and their positive effects for the whole community. It mobilises social support for the project, and facilitates active participation in the implementation of concrete actions.

Personnel involved in the LAP noted a decline in the number of active participants in the project from several dozen people at the beginning to a dozen in the final stage of the project. Initially, participation was associated with the implementation of socially useful assigned work, and with the possibility of earning some extra money. Later, when these opportunities ended, a much smaller number of people engaged in cultural and educational activities carried out by the animators. The animators emphasised that the involvement of broader groups of inhabitants in the activities was very limited, and usually restricted to passive participation.

According to the animators, greater involvement of the wider community, not just those who signed the contract, would be more likely if the project were based on local leaders, if there were any local leaders. However, the residents said that in their community it was difficult to identify people who by most, or even some, inhabitants were considered to be leaders. In addition, people who were more involved and could pretend to a leadership role were often negatively perceived by other community members.

> "I have got involved very heavily in this project. I encourage people to come to jointly act, do something together, because it is for all of us. They answered me that I probably get paid for it, or that I do get involved to get something special from the social welfare centre. Then I said that it does not make sense." (A woman of 55, a resident of Kaufhaus)

It is also worth noting that in the case of the LAP in Kaufhaus there was an attempt to create a 'local leader' by exposing the most active participant.

> "At the beginning they invited me, met with me, at festivities I performed on stage, the mayor shook my hand. And then as I spoke a couple of times that something did

> not fit to me, it's not so!" (A woman of 55, a resident of Kaufhaus)

The project animators also emphasised that the initial cooperation with the person presented as a local leader was very good. Unfortunately, this changed later on. In their view, the 'local leader' had more and more demands and became unmanageable.

> "The lady at the beginning was the main driving force behind this part of the community that wanted to do something. At the beginning there was great cooperation – she encouraged everyone to action, but later mistook her roles. She wanted to determine, manage people and workers, wanted to be smarter than the head of the centre." (Employee of local welfare centre)

The main dilemma when trying to activate peoples' social potential and empower community leadership is the possibility of a situation in which the goals of local leaders diverge from the project objectives. In such a situation it is necessary to conduct a mediation process to sustain cooperation. Lack of agreement may lead to conflict not only between implementers of the project and a leader, but also with a significant part of the community. In the Kaufhaus case the leadership potential was wasted, and with it the opportunity to build on the cooperation with existing leaders of the local community. However, strong social capital, together with the involvement of a leader of the community, seems to provide a fruitful base for local development. This probably requires greater autonomy in the operation of community, which is difficult to achieve when the institution implementing the project plays such a key role.

Conclusion

The Kaufhaus local community is beset by several problems: a high degree of social disintegration, a very low level, even a lack, of social capital (which could be used to undertake actions to activate the whole community), a high degree of poverty and multiple social problems. About 50% of the households rely on support from the social welfare centre. The inhabitants lack trust in the local authority, resulting in a lack of willingness to cooperate. They also display negative attitudes to social welfare institutions. All these factors make it difficult, and in some cases impossible, to achieve the objectives of the project.

In addition, attention should be drawn to some mistakes that were made during the planning and implementation of the project and ultimately led to difficulties in achieving expectations:

- Given the specificity of the community and attitudes to local authorities and social aid institutions, sufficient efforts was not taken to involve inhabitants in the planning and implementation of activities.
- The diagnosis of social problems, determination of needs, and resulting goals of the project were based on expert knowledge and analyses of existing data, not on cooperative agreement with members or representatives of the community.
- The activities undertaken mainly focused on social welfare clients and did not activate wider social groups to a sufficient extent.
- Although the project introduced reasonably well-developed tools for the social integration of people at risk of social exclusion, most of the people involved did not fall into this category.

Nevertheless, it should be noted that the LAP actually gave some members of the community an opportunity to undertake socially useful assigned work, and established a group of people who for some years were actively involved in the project. This group is relatively small, but it could serve as the foundation for the activation of other members of the community and the creation of social capital within it. So far this group has mainly concentrated on internal integration, internal cultural and educational development a. It would be beneficial for the community if this group were to focus more on involving the wider community in solving common problems and tackling community needs in collaboration with local institutions, organisations and authorities.

The lesson to be drawn from the Kaufhaus case is that the process of designing activities of broadly defined local community organising should be based on serious consultation and dialogue between the public authority that is usually the initiator of such activities and the subordinate institutions that carry out these activities. By doing so one can achieve the following:

- A better understanding of citizens' needs and problems, and thus a chance to satisfy needs and solve problems. Community members know best their needs and how they feel about their problems. If they were allowed to articulate them, it would be easier to design projects to target factual (not imagined) needs and problems. The effects would presumably be more satisfying for the residents, encouraging them to get involved in project activities.

- More precise determination of priorities of action. This is crucial for better allocation of available resources. Financial resources are always limited and insufficient. Social consultations allow for creating a list of priorities accepted by the community, thereby preventing unnecessary tensions and misunderstandings. This is how participatory budgets operate (see Ganuza and Baiocchi, 2012; Sintomer et al, 2012; Kłębowski 2013).
- Better information provision to prospective participants, which prevents surprise and negative reactions when activities are initiated. When the purpose is not clear enough or fully understood, there is a risk of opposition. In particular, the failure to communicate and give adequate warning about temporary difficulties and complications arising from the activities of local community organising (such as repair work to infrastructure) can trigger opposition. Community members have to fully understand and anticipate the effect of such activities to endure the discomfort;
- Quick feedback on emerging problems before they take proportions that disturb social peace. The consultation of planned activities provides an opportunity to examine the reaction of community members to the proposed objectives of the project. This is particularly important in situations when some elements of a project are controversial and evoke strong opposition at the planning stage. Consultations provide an opportunity to prepare an alternative solution, which will help to avoid tensions, conflicts, and sometimes even open protest.
- An increase in citizens' trust in the authorities and support for their activities in the future. Local authorities have much to gain if they approach members of the community in the reciprocal manner of partnership. Such spirit of partnership allows for decisions that have direct meaning to citizens. This will in turn increase the legitimacy of the local authority and make the citizens more open for future cooperation (see also Długosz and Wygnański, 2005).

Projects that empower residents not only create social ties and encourage the pursuit of common goals and shared problem solving, but also shape a willingness to cooperate, and a tendency to learn, take responsibility and perpetuate patterns of social and civic activism. It is important that at the outset such projects rely on both the knowledge of experts and professionals and the opinions of residents, who often have the best understanding of their needs and problems.

Through dialogue with the community it is possible to find other important elements shaping the actions and aspirations of community members. Such elements include, for example, the value residents assign to particular spatial elements that create a feeling of 'being home'. Such spatial elements can be the spaces of everyday life, work, upbringing and so on. Through dialogue we get to know people's motivations, values and norms, and the importance of local tradition and history, thus facilitating mutual understanding.

Local community organising should involve citizens from the outset of the project until its final evaluation in joint activities aimed at changing unfavourable circumstances. Citizens' participation in actions, whether related to funding or decision making, whether actual or ideational, results in their activation, thus building a sense of belonging and responsibility for the implementation and results of the project.

Notes

1. Based on results from the international research project SPHERE, financed within European Union's Seventh Framework Programme. The Polish research team was led by Professor Kazimiera Wódz.
2. 'Civil dialogue' or 'civil society dialogue' is, to some extent, a structured format for public dialogue that provides a tool to build bridges across the chasm of public viewpoints and opinions, especially regarding controversial topics. Civil dialogue is sometimes used by official institutions like the European Commission in its Europe for Citizens Programme. It is also used to form regional policies within the European Union, including in Ruda Śląska. Social work in parts of Poland rely on the civil dialogue tool, which is also studied by Polish social work researchers (see, for example, Mandrysz 2007).
3. Expertise: Local Activities Programs as instruments of activation of the local community in solving the residents' problems: K. Wódz, K. Faliszek, B. Kowalczyk, E. Leśniak-Berek, W. Mandrysz. Katowice 2008.

References

Cohen, M. (1978) 'Community organization and illustration of practice', in A. Fink (ed) *The field of social work* (7th edn), New York, NY: Holt, Rinehart and Winston.

Cox, F.M., Erlich, J.L., Rothman, J. and J. E. Tropman (eds) (1987) *Strategies of community organization* (4th edn), Itasca: F.E. Peacock Publishers Inc.

Długosz, D. and Wygnański, J.J. (2005) *Obywatele współdecydują. Przewodnik po partycypacji społecznej* [Citizens co-decide. Guide to social participation], Warszawa: Forum Inicjatyw Pozarządowych.

Ecklein, J. and Lauffer, A. (1971) *Community organizers and social planners*, New York, NY: Wiley and Sons.

Ganuza, E. and Baiocchi G. (2012) 'The power of ambiguity: how participatory budgeting travels the globe', *Journal of Public Deliberation*, 8(2): 1-12.

Giza-Poleszczuk, A. and Hausner J. (eds) (2008) *The social economy in Poland: Achievements, barriers to growth, and potential in light of research results*, Warsaw: Foundation for Social and Economic Initiatives.

Haynes, K. and Holmes, K. (1994) *Invitation to social work*, New York, NY: Longman.

Kaźmierczak, T. and Rymsza, M. (eds) (2007) *Kapitał społeczny. Ekonomia społeczna* [Social capital. Social economy], Warszawa: Instytut Spraw Publicznych.

Kłębowski, W. (2013) *Budżet partycypacyjny. Krótka instrukcja obsługi* [Participatory budgeting. Short manual], Warszawa: Instytut Obywatelski.

Mandrysz, W. (2007) *Znaczenie dialogu obywatelskiego dla kształtowania polityki regionalnej Województwa Śląskiego na tle polityki spójności Unii Europejskiej* [The importance of civil dialogue in shaping regional policy Province of Silesia on the background of European Union cohesion policy], Katowice: Uniwersytet Śląski Wydział Nauk Społecznych, Instytut Socjologii.

Mayo, M. (1994) 'Community work', in C. Hanvey and T. Philpot (eds) *Practising social work*, London: Routledge, pp 67-79.

Mayo, M. (1998) 'Community work', in R. Adams, L. Dominelli and M. Payne (eds) *Social work. Themes, issues and critical debates*, Basingstoke: Macmillan, pp 160-72.

McLaughlin, K., Osborne, S.P. and Ferlie, E. (2002) *New Public Management: Current trends and future prospects*, London: Routledge.

Payne, M. (2005) *Modern social work theory* (3rd edn), Basingstoke and New York, NY: Palgrave Macmillan.

Ross, M. (1967) *Community organization: Theory, principles and practice*, New York, NY: Harper and Row Publishers.

Rothman, J. and Tropman, J.E. (1987) 'Models of community organization and macro practice perspectives: their mixing and phasing', in F.M. Cox, J.L. Erlich, J. Rothman and J.E. Tropman (eds) *Strategies of community organization* (4th edn), Itasca: F.E. Peacock Publishers Inc.

Sintomer, Y. H.C., Röcke, A. and Allegretti, G.(2012) 'Transnational models of citizen participation: the case of participatory budgeting', *Journal of Public Deliberation*, 8(2): 1-32.

Twelvetrees, A. (2008) *Community work* (4th ed), New York, NY: Palgrave Macmillan. Weil, M. (2005) *The handbook of community practice*, Thousand Oaks, CA: Sage Publications.

Wódz, K. (1998) *Praca socjalna w środowisku zamieszkania* [Social work in the living environment], Katowice: Wydawnictwo Śląsk.

Wódz, K. and Kowalczyk, B. (2014) *Organizowanie społeczności. Modele i strategie działania* [Organizing the community. Models and strategies], Warszawa: Centrum Rozwoju Zasobów Ludzkich.

Part 4
Assessment, negotiation and decision making

THIRTEEN

On the unnoticed aspects of professional practice

Rasmus Antoft, Kjeld Høgsbro, Maria Appel Nissen and Søren Peter Olesen

Introduction

In the policy for implementation of the Social Investment Package of the European Commission 2013-14, European welfare states were encouraged to invest in welfare and to reform welfare states. It was emphasised how they should 'streamline governance and reporting' with a focus on 'monitoring financial, economic and social outcomes', and 'building evidence based knowledge and policy' (European Commission, 2013). Denmark seems to comply with these discourses of governance. Currently, the prevailing ideas of governing and reforming welfare services are focused on so-called evidence-based research (EBR), policy and practice (EBP) (Hansen and Rieper, 2010; Høgsbro, 2010). For example, the National Board of Social Services promotes a combination of evidence-based methods, systematic knowledge production, and cost-benefit and cost-effectiveness analysis to be implemented in practice (Nissen, 2015). In Denmark, there has not yet been a comprehensive and coherent research programme exploring the consequences of this form of governance. Albeit it is assumed that EBR and EBP will improve welfare services, there is currently no evidence that it will in fact enhance quality and accountability in professional practice. On the contrary, a major critique of EBR and EBP is that the inevitable contextual conditions of welfare services and the complexities of professional practices are ignored (Pawson, 2006).

Professional practice is dependent on the capacity to perform professional discretion in complex contexts and situations dealing with ambiguous problems, which do not prescribe a certain solution. Within this realm it becomes extremely important that professionals have the capability to act with constant care. This capacity to deal with what is *not* evident is often considered a constitutive element of professional practice (Grimen, 2008). If this inherent ambiguity of professional practice goes unnoticed, there is a risk that efforts to streamline performance will be counterproductive, because it would not facilitate, and in worst case would undermine, professional discretion. Accordingly, the aim of this chapter is to make visible some important aspects of professional practice that go unnoticed in the realm of EBR and EBP. We show how professional practice is far from streamlined *due to* contextual and situational complexities – and how in particular negotiation in 'fuzzy' realities, reflection on risks and cooperation despite controversies are crucial in terms of handling these ambiguities. We do that progressively throughout the chapter, providing an analysis of cases, each and together illustrating this point. The cases derive from a collection of Danish qualitative research projects, each concerned with professional practice. At the end of the chapter, we discuss the implications of the analysis for research and professional development.

Negotiation in 'fuzzy' realities

The concept of negotiations is a metaphor for what takes place in interactions between actors in a specific social setting (Levin and Trost, 2005). According to Anselm Strauss, whenever or wherever professionals interact to organise professional work practices and shared tasks, negotiations occur. Negotiations often occur when rules and policies for practice are not inclusive, when there are disagreements between professionals, when there is uncertainty and when change is introduced (Strauss, 1978). When social order – the shared agreements, the binding contracts that constitute the grounds for an expected, non-surprising, taken-for-granted, even ruled orderliness of everyday practice – is disturbed, parties will attempt to create a negotiated order enabling shared work tasks to be solved. These negotiations unfold in arenas of work practice contextualised in specific organisational and interprofessional settings, and they often function as unnoticed practices of day-to day routines of organising professional work. Andrew Abbott defines such social arenas as 'fuzzy' realities in which a number of issues are at stake for the involved professionals (Abbott, 1988). In such settings, professional boundaries are crossed and become fluid, compromises are made, and negotiations on the right theories and methods for problem solving unfold. The following example is an illustration of this.

An informal and strategic endeavour

The following example of negotiations in a fuzzy reality derives from a field study on power and negotiations in interprofessional relations (Antoft, 2005).[1] The study focused on the micro processes of diagnostic work on people with symptoms of dementia. By analysing interactions between municipality dementia nurses, general practitioners, hospital nurses and doctors in the arenas of shared diagnostic work, the study showed that processes of negotiation were not just about getting the work done, but also about setting the boundaries for gaining control of or giving up professional ('dirty') work. Dirty work refers to tasks that are viewed as physically, socially or morally tainted (Hughes, 1971), and as a consequence are less attractive to the professional's aspiration for professional status and identity. The following case exemplifies how dementia nurses and GPs interact and strategically negotiate how diagnostic work should be done.

The scene for this case is the investigation of an elderly woman of 89 years, who is suspected to be suffering from dementia. The patient is struggling with other diseases, including depression and possible colon cancer. The starting point of the diagnostic work is the Aalborg Municipality dementia assessment model and its formal guidelines for diagnostic tools and division of labour between dementia nurses and GPs. Yet there is no agreement between the parties as to the right time to stop the diagnostic process, and be satisfied with the investigation result. Following the dementia assessment model, the GP makes an initial diagnosis of the elderly woman's condition and contacts the dementia nurse to initiate cooperation on investigation of dementia symptoms. After examination and diagnosis of the patient's symptoms, the GP decides that it is not appropriate to send the patient on to a CT scan and further diagnostic work in the secondary sector. A CT scan and an examination by a specialist doctor at a hospital are the preconditions to medical treatment for dementia. The GP explains that he is aware of his power base, a position that allows him to dictate certain actions. But he stresses that the diagnostic process does not stop just because the GP can. It is based on a professional and personal assessment of what is in the patient's interest. Again, arguments relating to the patient's age and other potential diseases appear. But the GP's actions and decisions are not negotiable. When he decides that the diagnostic process should stop, his decision is non-negotiable. However, the nurse suggests what the GP should do in this particular case; the patient pathway should be completed with a referral to the secondary sector. Although the nurse is critical towards the GP's reasoning for not continuing the investigative work, she is still satisfied with the results of the work carried out. The doctor makes a written diagnosis that can be taken as a legitimate basis for a special follow-up with health and social care initiatives in the municipality. The dementia nurse withdraws from the conversation with the GP without further confrontation. She does not try to convince or persuade the GP to continue the assessment project. It is accepted that it is the doctor's decision and that he sets the premise for collaborative work and potential negotiations in this specific patient pathway.

Negotiating processes takes different forms. In this specific case, the GP sets the agenda for the shared diagnostic work and obtains a non-bargaining position, where the nurse's role is defined by the GP's position in the professional hierarchy and his ability to set the agenda. The GP's knowledge of the patient's multiple diseases and everyday life situations becomes decisive. But the nurse's strategy changes during the process. As the GP stops the patient pathway, even though the nurse disagrees with the decision, she withdraws from the negotiating arena, since the diagnostic work being done will enable future work with the patient within the municipality.

However, the nurse's narrative entails another interesting strategy for pursuing the agenda of the municipality and her profession. In other cases, where the GP for multiple reasons does not wish to engage in collaborative work on diagnosing patients with symptoms of dementia, the municipality has adopted a practice whereby dementia nurses are given the authority to make a preliminary diagnosis based on their specialist knowledge and tools for assessing symptoms of dementia. As a consequence, the diagnostic work becomes a cross-boundary activity in which the formal division of labour between doctors and nurses becomes fuzzy. In cases of dementia, this practice was often accepted by the GP, since this type of psychiatric diagnosis and work with demented people was considered dirty work. There is no treatment for the disease, only for the symptoms, and dealing with the patients and their families was time-consuming and considered by some GPS to be a nuisance, and, as a consequence, dirty work.

The example here illustrates how professional practices are characterised by informal negotiating processes and strategic action, and that the outcome of these processes depends both on position in the division of labour – the shadow of hierarchy – and on the professional knowledge and judgement applied in the diagnostic process. The result of such processes is not necessarily agreement on the right model for problem solving, and a logically rational connection between goals and actions might not exist (see, for example, Svensson, 1996; Allen, 1997). This becomes even clearer in the following case.

A conversational, linguistic and dynamic process

The next example further emphasises the informal negotiated character of professional decision making by addressing the details of language use in institutional practice. The excerpt derives from a meeting concerning the residual working capability of a client, who has worked for 17 years as laboratory technician, which has led to constant pains in her neck, shoulder and arms.[2] It is taken from a study of employment-oriented social work, demonstrating interprofessional interaction at a Danish jobcentre.[3] The professionals – two caseworkers and a medical consultant – use different types of knowledge, discussing the future of a client, who has been declared to have no remaining working ability. They are drawing on common sense and caseworker experience as well as knowledge from the social and medical sciences in delicate negotiations, thus displaying competing versions of the client's situation. They even try to present themselves as accountable (Eskelinen et al, 2008), and, having reached a conclusion, join in a rationalisation of the decision made. Both the colleague and the medical consultant agree with the conclusion drawn by the caseworker in charge based on statements made by the rehabilitation centre concerning the clients working capability. But although they agree with the conclusion they do not relinquish their position or arguments entirely, but add 'accounts' – explanations, justifications and excuses (see also Scott and Lyman, 1968) – for their consent, for example by referring to consequences, and the lack of lenient jobs available and alternatives in general. This means that decisions are not obtained as a rational choice between alternatives. Rather, it seems as if decisions are constructed as inevitable conclusions that need to be explained afterwards. Furthermore, processes rather than decisions as such become visible when looking into the 'black box' of professional practice (Boden, 1994).

25:30	SA1	"... but if the damage has occurred in her shoulder and arms ..."
25:33	SA2	"Well, I can see that, but how is she managing at home then, I think.... I don't believe that she doesn't do anything at all <no>, that she is sitting in a chair <no> with armrests, and then she is just sitting there ..."
25:46	SA1	"I don't believe that either, because that's not the way she is. She is actually more like ..."
25:50	SA2	"I, I can't understand, if she is not capable of managing something alternating ... I can't understand that <no>."
26:10	LK	"Well, these people, who are very perfectionistic and put big demands on themselves, they have really problems when they get a health problem, because then they don't feel – they are just like 'on-off' or 'either-or' <yes, yes>, so, if they can't deliver 100%, then it's no good <no> ..."
26:27	SA2	"No, but still ..."
26:29	LK	"And if you work a little with this experience related to performing a piece of work, then it might be, you might move some way, but it needs to be done that piece of work."
26:38	SA1	"Yes, that's just what the rehabilitation cen ... <yes>"
26:42	SA2	"Yes, but just make a pot of coffee once or twice ..."
26:46	SA1	"Yes, but it isn't ..."
26:49	SA2	"We can put forward some suggestions as regards, what we believe, she can, whether we can find it or not ..."
26:57	LK	"Then she is on unemployment benefit, yes. But the question is whether the process has taken place inside her head <yes>. We don't know that."

The excerpt shows how competing versions of categorisation of the client are put into play (25:30; 25:33; 26:57), how the discussion at a specific point tends to threaten the caseworker in charge (26:29; 26:38), and thus how negotiations are not simply discussions of matters of fact but include the face and the accountability of the professionals involved. Negotiating competing versions of categorisation of the client and rationalising a decision made, or, rather, a conclusion/consensus obtained, the excerpt demonstrates how participants soften their own argumentation without abandoning it, for instance when one of the participants says to the caseworker in charge (whose position is the one accepted in the conclusion) that she 'had no other choice under the circumstances'. Another way of doing this is by arguing that in principle the original suggestion is still valid, but may not realistic at this point in this case. Thus, even if her conclusion is contested, the caseworker in charge obtains consent from the other participants. The case indicates how decision making appears to be a matter of negotiating competing versions of categorisation rather than a matter of medical diagnosis and choice of treatment. When it is not obvious which version to choose, there is a risk related to knowledge, as the next example shows.

Reflections on risk

In professional decision making, the process of obtaining knowledge cannot be reduced to a process of making rational choices between alternatives based on full information. On the contrary, professional practice is constantly challenged by both a 'surfeit' and a 'deficit' of knowledge (Von Oettingen, 2007): Professional practice is often overburdened by interactional complexity providing a surfeit of knowledge, while at the same time professionals face problems shrouded in genuine uncertainties and deficits in knowledge. In contrast to this, expectations of performance often appear discursively as 'necessities' with a reference to generalised assumptions about 'reality'. Professional practice is situated between these forms of knowledge, and the difficult task of reconciling them is at heart in many informal negotiations. What is at stake is the risk of ignorance: the possibility that at some point in the future, it will be recognised that certain forms of knowledge, which might have contributed to solving a problem, were not, but could have been, obtained. As such, the risk of not knowing and the need for reflection is a crucial element of professional practice. However, research has pointed out how expectations of performance combined with risk awareness can be counterproductive. Standardised forms of risk assessment based on generalised knowledge are often introduced for the purpose of minimising the risk of ignorance, to promote safety and prevent harm. However, there is also a risk that such standardised efforts do not work as expected if they undermine the space for professional discretion and reflection (Taylor and White, 2006; Broadhurst et al, 2010; Munro, 2011). The following case from child welfare exemplifies this by showing how general expectations in relation to risk assessment can interact with and lead to problems of reflection and professional discretion (Nissen, 2005, 2006).[4]

A mother with an addiction to unspecified pills and hash is pregnant. The caseworker worries, but since the mother expresses a willingness to stop smoking hash and is looking forward to becoming a mother, she refers the mother and her new-born child to a 24-hour family treatment institution. The purpose is to investigate and assess her parental skills. At the institution, professionals use a standardised model for systematic assessment. However, they find it difficult to get a picture of the parental skills of the mother mainly because the mother

> is reluctant to participate in the everyday activities of the institution. Some of the professionals start to worry. They think the mother is isolating herself and the child. They find her reasons for not participating in everyday activities 'strange' and 'paranoid'. They wonder if there is something 'psychiatric' at play, and address the risk of not being able to observe the mother; they might overlook something important. Other professionals, assigned as the mother's contact persons, assess the mother differently. They emphasise the mother's need for care and parental skills training. They propose a motivating strategy combined with close observations. At an assessment meeting among the professionals, divergent experiences of the mother and her behaviour are discussed. Despite alternative perceptions of the interactional complexity, the growing risk awareness among some of the professionals becomes decisive. Consequently, it is decided that the mother should be forced to participate in everyday activities and should not be allowed to leave the institution at weekends. It is also decided that the mother should undergo a neurological investigation to find out if her capability to learn has been harmed. This assessment is later conveyed at a meeting with the mother, the contact persons and the caseworker. At this meeting, both the mother and the caseworker question the knowledge of the professionals. The mother questions the professionals' capability of knowing the child's needs, given the fact that the child is still a baby. The caseworker questions the professionals' knowledge of substance abuse and challenges related to becoming 'clean'. She implies that they have not initiated the right treatment – professional counselling. In addition, she emphasises how treatment should not be about changing the mother's personality and preference for being a 'loner'. In light of this, the contact persons abandon the institutional agenda and accept the agenda of the caseworker.

This example illustrates how professionals are situated between the experience of interactional complexity in everyday practice and expectations of performance related to the assessment of parental skills. Situated in this position, the professionals are extremely aware of the risk of ignorance. This risk awareness and orientation towards expectations of performance create a process that may be counterproductive to reflection. Professional work is inevitably challenged by both a surfeit and a deficit in knowledge. This problem can only be handled through reflection, by embracing the inherent uncertainty of professional knowledge, and by recognising the problems of obtaining 'true' knowledge. An increase in risk awareness combined with high expectations of performance in relation to risk assessment can undermine this. Streamlining professional knowledge to avoid uncertainty does not reduce risk; rather it hinders reflection and increases the risk of ignorance. A major problem within this process is the reluctance to address and explore controversies in a cooperative way, which is the theme of our final example.

Cooperation despite controversy

Rational explanations legitimising professional interventions are crucial to professionals. This seems to be particularly urgent when legitimising interventions in the lives of people who are not supposed to be able to take care of their own interests (Høgsbro, 2002, 2010). Services cannot be legitimised by reference to the satisfaction of users deemed unable to take care of own interests and partly unable to understand their own situation. But the international discourses of disability are not unambiguous, and accordingly, they might become a point of departure for internal controversies and intense discussions among the professionals loaded with anger, confusion and ambivalence. To be responsible for the situation and the possible future of people in extremely vulnerable situations calls for a professional commitment where failures and questions of professional as well as personal responsibility and identity are of great concern. Research has revealed strange and unexpected examples of these ambiguities in advanced rehabilitation programmes for people with schizophrenia, drug abuse, autism, attention deficit hyperactivity disorder (ADHD) and traumatic brain injuries (Høgsbro, 2002, 2007, 2010; Høgsbro et al, 2003, 2012, 2013). The following case concerned with training programmes for preschool children may serve as an example (Høgsbro, 2007):[5]

> In the evaluation of training programmes for preschool children with autism, parents as well as professionals were identified as referring to two different discourses. One emphasised a caring and protecting environment that guarded the children from demands they could not live up to, and the other emphasised daily challenges that could develop their competences. Both discourses referred to UN conventions on disability rights saying that member states had to enhance the possibilities of people with disability so they could be on equal terms with ordinary people. But the first discourse understood this as being accepted on own terms and the other discourse understood it as being offered the best training possible that could help them meet 'normal' standards. The first discourse regarded the second as leading to the loss of self-respect, and the second regarded the first discourse as leading to segregation. Both regarded the other as breaking with the UN standard and ignoring the wellbeing and future perspective of the children. Both referred to a huge body of international research literature on autism. The conflict was loaded with feelings that touched the identity and responsibility of both parents and professionals. In their daily

practice the professionals asked themselves if they were actually betraying the children when accepting their deviance or if they were causing them stress by making too many demands. The parents asked themselves if they were depriving their children of opportunities in the future by accepting special education for people with autism, or if they would alternatively deprive them of happiness and self-respect by choosing an ordinary school with all the inherent pressure and social competition among ordinary children. Both groups were seeking information on the internet and were well informed about conflicting theories and research findings in the field.

This example shows how deeply discourses and professional conflicts, identity and ethics are interwoven, involving feelings such as professional dignity, self-respect and issues of legitimacy. Similar examples could be taken from brain injury rehabilitation as well as services offered to people with dementia, drug abuse, schizophrenia, ADHD and so forth. In every one of these fields, different discourses support different models of intervention and rehabilitation.

Some of the main arguments for EBR and EBP are related to these serious controversies within the professional world. Professionals, users, politicians and decision makers on all levels are looking for research that might reduce risk and put an end to controversies. But as our example shows, professional practice addresses individual circumstances and specific contexts and settings to a degree that demands cooperation and negotiated judgements built on the experiences of the actors involved. In these instances, EBR is only one of several sources. Dialogue and cooperation among professionals and users are equally important. Disagreements must be made visible and thus easier to tackle, and standardised concepts of rehabilitation and aid have to be adjusted to local and individual contexts. This does not eliminate risk, but enables the development of professional discourses.

Conclusion and implications for professional development

Whenever or wherever professionals interact to organise professional work practices and shared tasks, negotiations occur. These negotiations unfold in arenas contextualised in specific organisational and interprofessional settings, and they often function as unnoticed practices of the day-to day routines of organising professional work. Although unnoticed in the discourses of EBR and EBP, our analysis shows it is possible to explore such negotiations – for example by using ethnomethodological and conversation analytical approaches enabling us to 'look inside professional practice' (Hall and White,

2005; Olesen, 2005, 2012) to discover the 'invisible trade' (Pithouse, 1987) and to identify activities and language use in the shaping of interprofessional cooperation and boundary work, decision making and rationalisation (Hall et al, 2013). Our analysis also suggests that we pay attention to reflections on risk as an inevitable aspect of professional practice in modern society (Beck, 1992; Luhmann, 1993; Warner and Sharland, 2010). It is important to explore the relationship between governmental attempts to prevent failure and the space for both professional reflection and discretion. Finally, the analysis implies that strong and generalised discourses may lead to deeper conflict and ambivalence, stress and confusion among professionals, if they are not identified and explicitly understood as collective dilemmas and controversies. If the controversies are made visible through dialogue and cooperation, they can be used to develop professional self-respect, pride, identity and means of orientation and can create the means for adjusting interventions. Systematic reviews and means of accreditation ('streaming performance') are addressing these issues in a formal centralised way that should move the psychological strain on front-line professionals to a level of professional, scientific and political decisions based on 'evidence' (Høgsbro, 2013). But simultaneously the complex preconditions for professional practice and discretion go unnoticed. Recognising the unnoticed aspects of practice – negotiations in 'fuzzy' realties, reflection on risk, and cooperation despite controversies – may lead to a more informal and decentralised approach to professional development. However, it would include how professional practice actually works and would emphasise procedural transparency, aims, reasons and shared knowledge rather than compliance to scientifically legitimised forms of practice. It would make visible the conditions that enable professionals to act with constant care in everyday situations.

Notes

1 The example is from a PhD dissertation. The study was conducted in 2002-04 as a qualitative single case study based on observations of interprofessional encounters, focus and single interviews with health professionals and document studies on patient journals, policy documents and so on.

2 The excerpt includes about one minute of meeting talk with a few omissions marked with an ellipsis ; <> indicates feedback from other participants; the numbers in the first column are minutes and seconds from the beginning of the talk, which lasted about 40 minutes. SA1 is the caseworker in charge; SA2 is her colleague. Both are trained social workers. LK is a medical consultant from another organisation.

3 The study was based on observations, sound recordings of encounters and meetings, interviews and documents collected during a joint one-week stay at a Danish jobcentre in the spring of 2005, repeated in the autumn of the same year.

[4] The example derives from a qualitative comparative field study in two 24-hour family treatment institutions. The study was a part of a PhD project exploring programmes and professional practices in relation to assessment and decision making.

[5] The example derives from an evaluation of rehabilitation and training programmes for preschool children following either principles of Applied Behavior Analysis or the TEACCH-inspired (Treatment and Education of Autistic and Related Communications Handicapped Children) ordinary Danish training programmes. The evaluation comprised observations, interviews, psychological tests and questionnaires emphasising both discourses and outcome of training.

References

Abbott, A. (1988) *The system of professions. An essay on the division of labor*, Chicago, IL: University of Chicago Press.

Allen, D. (1997) 'The nursing-medical boundary: a negotiated order?', *Sociology of Health and Illness*, 19(4): 498-520.

Antoft, R. (2005) *Demenshåndtering – magt og forhandling i interprofessionelle relationer* [Handling dementia. Power and negotiations in interprofessional relations], Aalborg: Aalborg University.

Beck, U. (1992) *Risk society. Towards a new modernity*, London: Sage Publications.

Boden, D. (1994) 'Agendas and arrangements: everyday negotiations in meetings', in A. Firth (ed) *The discourse of negotiation. Studies of language in the workplace*, Oxford: Pergamon, pp 63-99.

Broadhurst K., Hall, C., Wastell, D., White, S. and Pithouse, A. (2010) 'Risk, instrumentalism and the human project in social work: identifying the informal logics of risk management in children's statutory services', *British Journal of Social Work*, 40(4): 1046-64.

Eskelinen, L., Olesen, S.P. and Caswell, D. (2008) *Potentialer i socialt arbejde. Et konstruktivt blik på faglig praksis.* [Potentials in social work. A constructive glance at professional practice], Copenhagen: Hans Reitzels Forlag.

European Commission (2013) *Policy road map for the 2013-2014 implementation of the social investment package. Employment, social affairs and inclusion*, Brussels: Employment, Social Affairs and Inclusion.

Grimen, H. (2008) 'Profesjon og kundskab' [Profession and knowledge], in A. Molander and L.I. Terum (eds) *Profesjonsstudier* [Studies of professions], Oslo: Universitetsforlaget, pp 71-85.

Hall, C. and White, S. (2005) 'Looking inside professional practice. Discourse, narrative and ethnographic approaches to social work and counselling', *Qualitative Social Work*, 4(4): 379-90.

Hall, C., Juhila, K., Matarese, M. and van Nijnatten, C. (eds) (2013) *Analysing social work communication. Discourse in practice*, London: Routledge.

Hansen, H.F. and Rieper O. (2010) 'The politics of evidence-based policy-making. The case of Denmark', *German Policy Studies*, 6(2): 87-112.

Høgsbro K. (2002) *Rehabilitering af mennesker med traumatiske hjerneskader på Kolonien Filidelfia* [Rehabilitation of persons with traumatic brain injury at Kolonien Filadelfia Rehabilitation Centre], Copenhagen: AKF-Forlaget.

Høgsbro, K. (2007) *ETIBA. En forskningsbaseret evaluering af rehabiliterings- og træningsindsatsen for børn med autisme, herunder evaluering af behandlingsmetoden ABA (Applied Behavior Analysis)* [ETIBA. Evaluation of preschool programmes for children with autism spectrum disorders in Denmark, with particular emphasis on the trial of ABA method (Applied Behaviour Analysis)], Aarhus: Marselisborgcentret.

Høgsbro, K. (2010) 'SIMREB – towards a systematic inquiry into models for rehabilitation', *Scandinavian Journal of Disability Research*, 12(1): 1-18.

Høgsbro, K. (2013) 'Evidensbegrebet i styringsteknologisk perspektiv' [The concept of evidence in a governance technological perspective], in H. Wadskjær (ed) *Metermålssamfundet* [Measurement Society], Aalborg: Aalborg Universitetsforlag.

Høgsbro K., Bovbjerg, K.M., Hardman, L.S., Kirk, M. and Henriksen, J. (2003) *Skjulte livsverdener: En etnografisk undersøgelse af forholdene for mennesker med hjemløshed, misbrug og sindlidelse som problem* [Hidden life-worlds: An ethnographic study of the conditions of persons suffering from the problems of homelessness, substance abuse and mental illness], Copenhagen: AKF-forlaget.

Høgsbro K., Eskelinen, L., Fallov, M.A., Mejlvig, K. and Berger, N.P. (2012) *Når grænserne udfordres. Arbejdsbelastninger og pædagogiske udfordringer i specialpædagogiske boenheder* [When borders are challenged. Work load and special pedagogical challenges in residential accommodation], Copenhagen: AKF-forlaget.

Høgsbro, K., Eskelinen, L., Lundemark, M. and Permin Berger, N. (2013) *ADHD-problematikkens sociale aspekter* [The social aspects of the ADHD problematic], Aalborg: Aalborg University.

Levin, I. and Trost, J. (2005) 'Symbolsk interaktionisme – hverdagslivets samhandling' [Symbolic interaction – everyday interaction], in M.H. Jacobsen and S. Kristiansen (eds) *Hverdagslivet: Sociologier om det upåagtede* [Everyday life: Sociologies of the unnoticed], Copenhagen: Hans Reitzels Forlag.

Luhmann, N. (1993) *Risk – a sociological theory*, Berlin: De Gruyter.

Munro, E. (2011) *The Munro review on child protection: Final Report. A child centered system*, London: UK Department for Education.

Nissen, M.A. (2005) *Behandlerblikket: Om sociale problemers tilblivelse, intervention og forandring i socialt arbejde med familier og børn med udgangspunkt i analyser af behandlingskommunikation på døgninstitutioner for familiebehandling* [The eye of the treatment: On social problems, intervention and change in social work with families and children based on analysis of treatment communication in 24-hour family treatment institutions], Aalborg: Aalborg University.

Nissen, M.A. (2006) 'Risiko og refleksion i socialt arbejde med familier og børn' [Risk and reflection in social work with families and children], *Nordiske Udkast*, (1): 61-80.

Nissen, M.A. (2015) 'Viden om viden og kvalitet' [Knowledge about knowledge and quality], in M. Harder and M.A. Nissen (eds) *Socialt arbejde I en foranderlig verden* [Social work in a changing world], Copenhagen: Akademisk Forlag.

Olesen, S.P. (2005, 2014) 'Samtaleanalyse – hverdagslivets kategorisering og sekventialitet' [Conversation analysis – categorization and sequentiality in everyday life], in M.H. Jacobsen and S. Kristiansen (eds) *Hverdagsliv – Sociologier om det upåagtede* [Everyday life – Sociologies of the unnoticed], Copenhagen: Hans Reitzels Forlag.

Olesen, S.P. (2012) 'Samtaleanalyse som sociologisk forskningstilgang. Om at udforske rækkefølge, betydningsdannelse og kontekster i social interaktion' [Conversation analysis as a sociological research approach. Investigating sequentiality, meaning-making and contexts in social interaction], in M.H. Jacobsen and S.Q. Jensen (eds) *Kvalitative udfordringer* [Qualitative challenges], Copenhagen: Hans Reitzels Forlag.

Pawson, R. (2006) *Evidence-based policy. A realist perspective*, London: Sage Publications.

Pithouse, A. (1987) *Social work. The social organisation of an invisible trade*, Aldershot: Avebury

Scott, M.B. and Lyman, S.M. (1968) 'Accounts', *American Sociological Review*, 33(1): 46-62.

Strauss, A.L. (1978) *Negotiations: Varieties, contexts, processes and social order*, San Francisco, CA: Jossey-Bass.

Svensson, R. (1996) 'The interplay between doctors and nurses – a negotiated order perspective', *Sociology of Health and Illness*, 18(3): 379-98.

Taylor, C. and White, S. (2006) 'Knowledge and reasoning in social work: education for human judgement', *British Journal of Social Work*, 36(6): 937-56.

Von Oettingen, A. (1997) 'Pædagogiske handlingsteorier i difference mellem teori og praksis' [Pedagogical theories of action in the difference between theory and practice] in A. Von Oettingen and F. Wiedemann (eds) *Mellem teori og praksis. Aktuelle udfordringer for pædagogiske professioner og professionsuddannelser* [Between theory and practice. Contemporary challenges for pedagogical professions and professional education], Odense: Odense University Press.

Warner, J. and Sharland, E. (2010) 'Editorial: special issue on risk and social work', *British Journal of Social Work*, 40(4): 1035-45.

FOURTEEN

Can complexity in welfare professionals' work be handled with standardised professional knowledge?

Lars Evertsson, Björn Blom, Marek Perlinski and Devin Rexvid

Introduction

In order to reduce uncertainty and complexity, and to prevent or manage the emergence of problematic situations in professional work, many welfare professions have experienced increased expectations to standardise and evidence base their professional practice (Grimen and Terum, 2009; Morago, 2010; Rexvid et al, 2012). To overcome problematic situations, reduce complexity and achieve best practice (Reynolds, 2000; Grimen and Terum, 2009), non-medical professions such as social workers are expected to adopt and implement the principles that underpin evidence-based medicine.

But what are the sources of complexity, uncertainty and problematic situations? In research on professions, complexity in professional work is often discussed in relation to the professional body of knowledge, and the role and use of expert knowledge (Larson, 1977; Abbott, 1988; Johnson, 1993; Freidson, 2004; Molander and Terum, 2010; Svensson and Karlsson, 2008; Svensson and Evetts, 2010). There is a tendency to relate professional success, problems, mishaps and shortcomings to flaws and limitations in the professions' expert knowledge or how that expert knowledge is utilised (Abbott, 1988; Sackett et al, 1996; Sackett, 2000; Howitt and Armstrong, 1999; Sekimoto et al, 2006; Serour et al, 2009; Hasenfeld, 2010; Molander and Terum, 2010; Morago, 2010).

However, in this chapter we are going to argue that complexity and problematic situations in professional work can have other sources. More precisely, based on two empirical studies of social workers within Swedish social services, we are going to show how complexity and social workers' perception of problematic situations stem out of everyday encounter with clients and the way that the work is organised.

The troublesome work organisation

In a Swedish study social workers reported that the way their work was organised gave rise to problematic situations and disrupted their professional practice (Perlinski, 2010; Perlinski et al, 2012). Based on the social workers' description we have chosen to call them specialised professional rooms and multiple timetables. Specialised rooms refers to social workers' description of how the work organisation divides their professional practice on several 'hands', thereby spatially separating social workers working with the same client. Multiple timetables refer to social workers' notion that the work organisation put high demands on social workers to synchronise and coordinate their work. But before we take a closer look at the problems connected with specialised professional rooms and multiple timetables we will give a short presentation of how personal social services (PSS) in Sweden are organised.

Social work and welfare provision in Sweden is to a large extent part of the public sector and especially a responsibility for the municipalities. In Sweden, municipalities have an extensive and constitutionally guaranteed autonomy. Part of that autonomy is the political and financial responsibility for providing personal social services to their citizens. Social work and especially the PSS in Sweden are regulated by the Social Services Act (SFS 2001:453), which is a framework law with few concrete regulations. In addition, since 1992 the Local Government Act (SFS 1991:900) provides the municipalities with the freedom to decide how they want to organise the discharge of the mandatory duties of the municipality.

Consequently, there is a large degree of variation among the 290 Swedish municipalities' political and organisational models of PSS. However, all these models have certain features in common: they all consist of a political part that sets goals and decides budgets, an administrative and executive managerial part, and a professional part that works directly with clients. The professional part may be organised in a wide range of ways. However, in the past two decades there has been a clear trend of abandoning integrated/generic models and instead embracing specialisation – a movement that in fact echoes the past (Perlinski, 2010).

In Sweden and in many other countries, a strong tendency within social work is to divide the PSS into specialised units and functions.

This tendency is especially clear in larger municipalities (Doel, 1997; Bergmark and Lundström, 1998; Lundgren et al, 2009). Common motives are political demands for renewal and increased efficiency.

Until the 1960s, social workers in Sweden focused on symptoms and were divided in different fields: childcare, care for drug abusers and monetary benefits. Each of those fields also had separate legislation. During the 1960s and 1970s, the idea of working in a more holistic way was introduced, and the different fields were merged into more integrated and homogenous organisational forms. The integration of childcare, care for drug abusers and monetary benefits implied that all social workers were expected to handle all kinds of problems and types of tasks. Consequently, the professional discretion of the social workers' expanded significantly. However, about the same time the idea of holistic working and integrated organisations was questioned and criticised. Behind this change were new influences in the field of organisation, but more importantly were the professional strivings from the social workers. Seen from the social workers' perspective, the idea of holistic working and integrated organisations hampered social workers possibility to develop expert skills and to become an expert in relation to specific client groups or tasks. Since the 1980s, when the new integrated Social Services Act was introduced, we have once more witnessed the increasing division of the social work role into different functions, where individual social workers handle a relatively delimited part of the work task.

Today, the clearly predominant organisational form is some kind of specialisation, and often problem specialisation. This implies a professional specialisation and division of labour among social workers. Social workers within PSS often specialise in working with a specific problem, for instance drug abuse, monetary benefits or unemployment, or with a specific category of client, for instance children, youngsters or immigrants. In 1989 around 51% of Swedish municipalities had some form of specialised PSS, but in 2007 the number had increased to 93% (Lundgren et al, 2009).

Specialised professional rooms

As mentioned earlier, one effect of the problem-specialised work organisation was that social workers who worked with the same client, but with different aspects of the client's problems, got spatially separated from each other. Spatial separation should be interpreted broadly. In some cases, it meant that the social workers were located in different parts of the same building or even in different buildings.

Problem specialisation gave thus rise to what can be seen as specialised professional rooms in the sense of social workers working exclusively with certain social problems, and with no or little contact with social workers working on other specialised tasks. From the survey, we could see how social workers perceived this spatial separation as causing problem in their everyday professional practice. The problems that social workers attributed to the spatial separation of professional practice were related to issues regarding cooperation, coordination and responsibility for a specific client.

Working with the same client but in different specialised professional rooms make cooperation and information exchange pivotal. However, social workers expressed that the spatial separation made cooperation and communication problematic. Lack of cooperation and communication was not only seen as a problem for the social workers, but also for the clients, who sometimes did not know whom to turn to, or which social worker was responsible for their case. In the survey, social workers highlighted the fact that the specialised organisation was not conducive to cooperation since there were no organisational structures and routines for how to bridge the professional practice that was carried out in the different specialised professional rooms.

To be able to cooperate and to apply a holistic perspective to clients' problems and life situation information was seen a key factor. However, the social workers complained that spatial separation resulted in a failure to share important information. Social workers pointed out that their organisation was ill equipped to transfer information from one specialised room to another. Sometimes, the lack of organisational structures and routines could be overcome through informal personal contacts. However, informal sharing of information was sensitive to disruption since it rested on personal bonds and trust. One cause of disruption was that the lack of organisational capacity left social workers with little incentive to share information outside of their specialised rooms. In some instances, the lack of incentives gave rise to what some social workers called 'territorial marking' or 'territorial pissing', that is jealously marking, guarding and defending the own area of expertise, and keeping the information and knowledge they work with within their own specialised professional room.

The lack of formal structures supporting professional cooperation made it difficult for social workers to plan and undertake coordinated professional action. Social workers described how coordinated professional practice outside of the specialised professional rooms had an ad-hoc character due to unclear professional roles and leadership. Unclear professional roles and leadership reflected negatively on questions regarding responsibility. Social workers expressed that they could find themselves working with the same client without anyone being in charge of planning and coordinating the professional work.

Multiple timetables

Dividing professional practice into specialised professional rooms gave rise to yet another problem that hampered the ability to cooperate and coordinate professional practice. To be able to cooperate and to coordinate professional practice when working with the same client required the coordination of multiple timetables. However, this was difficult since it was often unclear who was responsible for developing a master timetable that would coordinate the many different timetables. In the absence of a master timetable, the work carried out in different specialised professional rooms was planned and set according to social workers' own specialised tasks. In the survey we could see that this coordination of different timetables was perceived as a problem, especially in those situations where working on a client's problem required the sequential linking of the different specialised professional rooms. However, social workers also expressed problems with synchronising their timetables in situations where clients' needs made in necessary to cooperate and coordinate professional practice in such a manner that they simultaneously worked with the client.

In this section we have shown that the most frequent model for organising professional social work in Sweden gives rise to problematic situations that do not reflect lack of professional knowledge or lack of professional competence. These situations do not constitute 'knowledge problems' and therefore cannot be solved by adding knowledge to social workers' professional knowledge base. Rather, the problems described can be seen as an unintended consequence of the specialised work organisation and the disruption it causes to professional practice.

Troublesome relationships with the client

In the previous section we showed that the way personal social services are organised may disrupt social workers' professional practice. We also argued that this disruption does not reflect lack of professional knowledge among social workers. In this section we give another example of disruption to social workers' professional practice. However, the focus here is on how everyday encounters with clients cause problems and disrupt social workers' professional practice.

The data consists of written narratives where social workers described situations that they perceived as problematic. Our preliminary assumption was that the narratives would reflect situations in which social workers experienced lack of knowledge, inability to set a correct diagnosis, or ambiguities regarding interventions or treatments. However, the narratives rarely touched on these issues. Rather, social workers described 'problematic situations' as situations where they felt that encounters with clients were disruptive to their professional practice.

In our data we were able to identify four different types of encounter that social workers perceived as disruptive to their professional practice. Common to these situations was that the clients hampered the social workers' professional work through displaying an unwillingness to participate or to change; making attempts to negotiate their client status; expressing a lack of motivation; or displaying a lack of trust in the social workers. Through their actions clients made it difficult for social workers to carry out fundamental aspects of professional work such as diagnostic work, needs assessment and selection of intervention and treatment (Hasenfeld, 1983, 2010; Abbott, 1988).

Unwilling clients

To be able to assess clients' needs and suggest appropriate intervention, social workers need information from the client. Situations were clients were unwilling to provide this information were therefore seen as problematic. Sometimes clients' unwillingness was overt in the sense that clients very openly chose not to share any information with the social worker and actively opposed any assessment or intervention. However, in most cases unwillingness had a covert character where clients tried to make themselves invisible or inaccessible to professional assessment and intervention. Clients did not show up to their appointments, did not keep agreements, refused to stay in contact with the professionals or restricted their contact to phone or email. Seen from the perspective of social workers, overt and covert resistance was experienced as undermining their professional authority and bringing their professional work to halt.

Bargaining clients

Clients who tried to set the agenda by bargaining were another source of disruption to social workers' professional practice. Through bargaining clients tried to gain a more favourable assessment or handpick preferable interventions and services. This made it hard for social workers to work in a systematic and structured way, especially in situations where social workers tried to follow standardised protocol or guidelines, or work in accordance with best practice or evidence-based practices.

Unmotivated clients

Situations where clients expressed lack of motivation were experienced as problematic by social workers since the clients' own driving force or initiative to change their current situation or lifestyle was identified as an important condition to successfully addressing and treating their problems. For social workers, clients' lack of motivation typically involved clients who did not want to engage in an assessment, pursue a treatment, or change a lavish consumption habit or unsatisfactory system of money management. To work with clients without motivation was challenging since most of the social workers' professional practice – methods and interventions – at least to some extent presupposed motivated clients.

Distrustful clients

Social workers perceived as problematic those situations where they felt that clients could not be trusted. Lack of trust was typically associated with clients behaving in a manipulative manner. Seen from the social workers' perspective, lack of trust introduced an element of uncertainty into their professional practice. This uncertainty made it harder to establish a clear picture of the clients' problems, assess their needs and choose an intervention. However, it was not only situations where clients behaved in a non-trustworthy way that were experienced as problematic. Social workers also perceived as problematic those situations where clients expressed a lack of trust and confidence towards them and their professional competence. Seen from the social workers' perspective, the absence of trust made it harder to gain information from the client and made some interventions less likely to work.

In this section we have shown how social workers' professional practice is ruptured by clients who exhibit resistance and act in a non-compliant way that neutralises their professional knowledge, methods and choice of interventions. According to Hasenfeld (1983), this is an inherent problem in human services organisations as the transformation of client attributes into organisational cases to some extent always requires cooperation and compliance on the client's part. Since lack of cooperation and compliance is an ever-present problem in professional practice, problems involving troublesome clients do not necessarily reflect lack of professional knowledge.

Discussion

Our two empirical cases represent problematic situations where the social workers' professional practice was ruptured, that is situations where social workers expressed difficulties maintaining a systematic and rational approach to professional work. In our cases, the rupture of professional practice was not a reflection of lack of knowledge or inadequate use of knowledge, nor could the problem be solved with more, alternative or better use of knowledge. Put another way, the problematic situations described in this chapter cannot be solved by standardised professional knowledge about interventions and results (Rose 1996; Power, 1997; Garsten et al, 2015). Attempts to solve the types of problematic situation described above by increasing or altering social workers' professional knowledge base would be a waste of resources since the rupture of professional practice derives from the way in which the work is formally organised and from everyday encounters with clients. In what follows we elaborate on why the problematic situations described in this chapter cannot be solved by focusing on the social workers' knowledge base.

As already mentioned, the predominant organisational form in Swedish PSS is problem-specialised work organisation. This is built on the assumption that the needs of the client can be broken down and separated into smaller pieces that can be 'treated' by functionally specialised social workers. This way of organising PSS has its merits, but based on the responses from our social workers it also has its drawbacks, especially in situations where social workers need to cooperate in order to meet the client's needs. The limitation of the problem-specialised work organisation becomes obvious in those situations where social workers have to transcend their specialised professional rooms and negotiate their individually set timetables in order professionally to address the client's problems. Seen from the perspective of our social workers, this adds to the complexity of their professional practice. However, this complexity is not primarily connected to the social workers' knowledge; rather, the complexity that is added to social workers' professional practice is purely organisational. Therefore, working with the social workers' knowledge base – screening instruments or evidence-based methods – or use of knowledge – manuals and so on – is likely to have no or little impact on this type of complexity. The complexity is the result of the way in which social work is organised within the problem-specialised work organisation:

- It is a complexity that originates from an organisational form where the 'average' client is assumed to be the bearer of social problems that are easily identifiable and for which interventions are readily available.
- It is an organisational form in which intra-professional cooperation, joint planning and coordination of interventions becomes a complex logistic challenge for social workers.

To improve the social workers' knowledge base or use of knowledge is also likely to be of limited use when professional practice is ruptured by clients who are unwilling to cooperate, lack motivation to change, try to negotiate, or act in a distrustful manner towards social workers. It is not the lack of, or use of knowledge, that makes these situation problematic. What makes situations like these problematic is the complexity that is added to social workers' professional practice when the relationship with the client does not permit them to establish or uphold a rational and systematic approach to their work. It hampers one or several central aspects of social workers' professional practice, for instance how to investigate and establish a client biography, assess the client's needs, plan and choose the proper intervention, or follow up the impact of intervention. It is a complexity that makes it difficult for social workers to establish a working timetable. It is hard to see how this kind of complexity could be tackled by addressing the social workers' knowledge base or use of knowledge, for instance by using checklists, manuals or evidence-based methods.

The role of knowledge in eradicating complexity in welfare professionals' work

For decades, knowledge and use of knowledge has had a central role in our understanding of professions and professional practice. There is a tendency to regard difficulties and problems in professional work mainly as an effect of the lack of formal knowledge or inability to use the right knowledge. Hence, welfare states invest considerable resources in raising professional groups' level of knowledge and in using evidence-based knowledge. And without doubt, lack of knowledge, the wrong kind of knowledge and erroneous knowledge use can induce problematic situations, which in turn can lead to perceptions of uncertainty and complexity. One of the main points in this chapter is, however, that experiences of uncertainty and complexity can have causes that are not related to knowledge at all, and that other 'solutions' may be more adequate. We argue that the notion of rational problem solving by using professional knowledge is hardly consistent with the fact that social work has an inherent complexity.

To express this more clearly, we draw on an analytical distinction between different types of tasks or problems, which is illuminating in this context. The social scientists Kim Forss, Mita Marra and Robert Schwartz (2011, p 15)[1] present a distinction between different types of tasks summarised in following three examples:

- The simple task – building a bridge. This is an engineering task and can be planned and executed in traditional blueprint format, and the evaluation afterwards is also a relatively simple task where handbooks and manuals can be followed.
- The complicated task – sending a rocket to the moon. Although an engineering task, this requires more and higher levels of expertise; there are no blueprints available. But rockets are similar and having sent one to the moon once increases the chance of success next time, and the outcome is highly certain.
- The complex task – raising a child. Raising one child provides experience but no assurance of success next time. The criteria of success differ and the outcome is variable, and you can never be certain of either. Every child is unique and there are no generally valid checklists for the task of evaluation.

Based on the distinction above, we conclude that the specialised social services are grounded on the assumption that social work deals with simple or complicated problems. This means that tasks are perceived as definable and clear, and that the social worker can be especially skilled and become a specialist within a certain area. To some extent, the social services obviously perform such tasks – take by way of example, short-term financial aid to people without other types of needs (simple problem), or an investigation of a foster home's appropriateness (complicated problem). Nonetheless, it is common for clients in contact with the social services to have significantly more complex problems that are often connected to their social position and situation. The issue is often a combination of problems, such as poverty, substance abuse, relationship problems, mental health problems, child abuse, and so on. Therefore, it is hardly controversial to say that social work within the social services largely involves working with complex problems. These kinds of multiple problem require tailored interventions adapted to individuals in unique situations. Such individually matched combinations of interventions are difficult to standardise and define in advance, and the results are seldom predictable.

As described earlier, some clients that social workers encounter in their daily work are perceived as problematic as they are unwilling or unmotivated, or attempt to bargain. We argue that such client encounters are typical examples of complex tasks, where the principal similarity with raising children is striking (see the earlier example from Forss et al [2015]). Manuals have limited application; helping one 'difficult' client provides experience but does not guarantee success with the next. Each client is unique and must be considered as an individual.

From our point of view, those responsible for the overall organisation and management of welfare professionals' work often neglect the element of complexity. Alternatively, they confuse complex tasks with complicated ones, and try to devise solutions designed either for simple or complicated problems, involving, for example, more standardisation or the use of evidence-based knowledge. We do not suggest that complexity is always impossible to handle, rather that it demand other solutions. If the answer to simple and complicated problems are specialised social services organisations, specific expertise and standardisation, complex problems demand organisations that enable flexible professional practice, general theoretical knowledge and situational adaptively.

We claim that there is an inherent and inevitable complexity in social work practice, and that efforts to reduce this complexity, with standardised professional knowledge, can lead to a paradox. That is, complexity could be perceived – by definition – as something negative that must be eliminated or reduced. This could imply that professionals, instead of trying to manage complexity in an adaptive and constructive way, limit their own opportunities to act by trying to avoid complexity.

A conclusion is that complexity in social work, and other welfare professions' work, can neither be avoided through organisational specialisation, nor eradicated by using standardised professional knowledge. Complexity must be addressed whether we want it or not. Instead of trying to avoid complexity and the uncertainty it brings, it is better to accept and approach it with open eyes. That increases the chances of finding constructive solutions that benefit clients as well as professionals.

Note

1 This distinction is based on a model proposed by Glouberman and Zimmerman (2002).

References

Abbott, A. (1988) *The system of professions. An essay on the division of expert labor*, Chicago, IL: University of Chicago Press.

Bergmark Å. and Lundström T. (1998) 'Metoder i socialt arbete: om insatser och arbetssätt i socialtjänstens individ- och familjeomsorg' [Methods in social work: an inventory analysis of practice in Swedish individual and family services], *Socialvetenskaplig Tidskrift*, 5(4): 291-314.

Doel, M. (1997) *Social work practice revisited: Generalist and specialist practice*, Occasional Monograph, Birmingham: Faculty of Health and Community Care, University of Central England.

Forss, K., Marra, M. and Schwartz, R. (eds) (2011) *Evaluating the complex: Attribution, contribution, and beyond*, New Brunswick, NJ: Transaction Publishers.

Freidson, E. (2004) *Professionalism. The third logic*, Cambridge: Polity Press.

Garsten, C., Lindvert, J. and Thedvall, R. (eds) (2015) *Makeshift work in a changing labour market: The Swedish model in the post-financial crisis era*, Cheltenham: Edward Elgar Publishing.

Glouberman, S. and Zimmerman, B. (2002) *Complicated and complex systems: What would successful reform of Medicare look like?*, Toronto: Commission on the Future of Health Care in Canada.

Grimen, H. and Terum, L (2009) *Evidensbasert profesjonsutøvelse* [Evidence-based professional practice], Oslo: Abstrakt Forlag.

Hasenfeld, Y. (1983) *Human service organizations*, Englewood Cliffs, NJ: Prentice-Hall.

Hasenfeld, Y. (2010) 'Worker-client relations: social policy in practice', in Y. Hasenfeld (ed) *Human services as complex organizations* (2nd edn), Los Angeles, CA: Sage Publications.

Howitt, A. and Armstrong, D. (1999) 'Implementing evidence based medicine in general practice: audit and qualitative study of antithrombotic treatment for atrial fibrillation', *British Medical Journal*, 318(7194): 1324-27.

Johnson, T.J. (1993) *Professions and power*, London: Macmillan.

Larson, M.S. (1977) *The rise of professionalism: A sociological analysis*, Berkeley, CA: University of California Press.

Lundgren, M., Blom, B., Morén, S. and Perlinski, M. (2009) 'Från integrering till specialisering – om organisering av socialtjänstens individ- och familjeomsorg 1988-2008' [From integration to specialisation: on the organising of personal social services 1998-2008], *Socialvetenskaplig Tidskrift*, 8(2): 162-83.

Molander, A. and Terum, L.I. (2010) 'Profesjonsstudier – en introduksjon' [Studying professional groups – an introduction], in A. Molander and L.I. Terum (eds) *Profesjonsstudier* [Studies of professions], Oslo: Universitetsforlaget.

Morago, P. (2010) 'Dissemination and implementation of evidence-based practice in the social services: a UK survey', *Journal of Evidence-Based Social Work*, 7(5): 452-65.

Perlinski, M. (2010) *Skilda världar – specialisering eller integration i socialtjänstens individ- och familjeomsorg* [Separate worlds – specialisation or integration in the personal social services], Umeå: Umeå University, Department of Social Work.

Perlinski, M. Blom, B. and Morén, S. (2012) 'Different worlds – different organisation models as conditions for working with clients in the Personal Social Services', *Social Work and Society*, 10(2): 1-18.

Power, M. (1997) *The audit society. Rituals of verification*, Oxford: Oxford University Press.

Reynolds, S. (2000) 'The anatomy of evidence-based practice: principles and methods', in L. Trinder and S. Reynolds (eds) *Evidence-based practice: A critical appraisal*, Oxford: Blackwell Science.

Rexvid, D., Blom, B., Evertsson, L. and Forssén, A. (2012) 'Risk reduction technologies in general practice and social work', *Professions and Professionalism*, 2(2): 1-18.

Rose, N. (1996) 'The death of the social? Re-figuring the territory of government', *International Journal of Human Resource Management*, 25(3): 327-56.

Sackett, D.L. (2000) *Evidence-based medicine*, Edinburgh: Churchill Livingstone.

Sackett, D.L., Rosenberg, W.M.C., Gray M.J.A., Haynes, B.R. and Richardson, S.W. (1996) 'Evidence based medicine: what it is and what it isn't', *British Medical Journal*, 312(7023): 71-2.

Sekimoto, M., Imanaka, Y., Kitano, N., Tatsuro, I. and Osamu, T. (2006) 'Why are physicians not persuaded by scientific evidence? A grounded theory interview study', *BMC Health Services Research*, 6(92).

Serour, M., Al Othman, H. and Al Khalifah, G. (2009) 'Difficult patients or difficult doctors: an analysis of problematic consultations', *European Journal of General Medicine*, 6(2): 87-93.

Svensson, L.G. and Evetts, J. (2010) *Sociology of professions: Continental and Anglo-Saxon traditions*, Göteborg: Daidalos.

Svensson, L.G. and Karlsson, A. (2008) 'Profesjoner og kontroll og ansvar' [Professions, control and responsibility], in A. Molander and L.I. Terum (eds) *Profesjonsstudier*, Oslo: Universitetsforlaget.

FIFTEEN

Who is viewed as client by social workers and general practitioners?

Devin Rexvid

Introduction

Welfare professions are described in different ways. A common way is to describe them as occupational groups that, on the basis of their specific mandate and their expertise, are considered to be best suited to solve citizens' problems and meet their needs (Molander and Terum, 2010; Svensson, 2010). However, a basic prerequisite for professionals to be able to solve problems and meet needs is that they clarify who has the problem or who can be considered as a client (Mosesson, 2000). Put differently, professions need to first figure out who is a client, in order to be able to initiate an intervention process that usually begins with diagnosis of the client's problem and generally ends with proposals for treating the problem (Hasenfeld, 1983; Abbott, 1988).

For many professions, the question of who is a client is self-evident or unproblematic. In research on professions and human services organisations it is often taken for granted that the person who pays for or seeks a service provided by professionals may be regarded as a client (Johnson, 1972; Hasenfeld, 1983; Abbott, 1988; Salonen, 2000). For professionals like social workers (SWs), however, this question is not so clear-cut, since a case can be initiated by persons other than the one who has a problem to be solved or a need to be met. More specifically, aside from individual clients, authorities or private individuals also can report to the social services a person who appears to be in need of the SWs intervention (Mosesson, 2000; Salonen, 2000). SWs are therefore often uncertain about who can be seen as a client. This chapter examines whom SWs and GPs view as a client, and how they gather information about the client and think about the client's problem. The data consists of vignette-based focus group interviews with 14 SWs and 11 GPs.[1] The chapter demonstrates that for SWs it is an initial and central element of their professional practice to identify who the client is, while for the GPs it is self-evident that the person who visits them with a problem is a client (the term client refers both to the clients met by SWs and the patients that GPs encounter in their professional practice). It is, however, important to point out that in certain cases it is the parent who takes a child to the doctor. In such a situation it is also obvious to the GP that it is the child, not the parent, that is the client.

The above-mentioned differences between SWs and GPs are important for our understanding of the factors that set the conditions for their professional practice. The findings in this chapter may be relevant to the attempts of policymakers and leaders in work organisations to reform or develop different professions' heterogeneous practice on the basis of homogenising programmes. The chapter also raises questions that may be of use in comparative studies of professions. Against this background, the purpose of this chapter is to describe and analyse how the question of who is seen as a client affects SWs' and GPs' professional practice. This is with particular reference to how professionals' perceptions of who is a client affects their professional practice in terms of gathering information, assessing information and information sources, and choosing an intervention.

In theoretical comparisons of SWs and GPs, the focus has often been on whether SWs meet the criteria that GPs fulfil, since the latter are regarded as archetypal professionals. In these comparisons, it is often professions' scientific knowledge base, status, monopoly and expertise that have been in focus (Brante, 2014; Brante et al, 2015; Dellgran, 2015). However, what professionals do in their practice and how they perform it has received less attention (Abbott, 1988; Dellgran, 2015).

In previous research on SWs' professional practice, considerable attention has been devoted to how SWs construct various types of clients or classify them into certain categories, such as problematic or voluntary clients. The focus of earlier research has thus been the consequences of SWs' performance of their professional practice for clients (Mosesson, 2000; Salonen, 2000; Järvinen, 2002; Järvinen and Mik-Meyer, 2003). The question of who is to be regarded as a client and what the answer to this question may mean for SWs' professional practice has gained little attention.

Neither has earlier research on GPs devoted much attention to the question of who they perceive as clients. One explanation for this is that most of GP clients voluntarily visit a GP for the problem they want help with (Freidson, 1961; Levin, 2013). This means that it is often clear to GPs whom they should regard as clients and relatively clear what the problem is and how it should be solved. That GPs often have a clear picture of who they regard as clients illustrates the conditions for exercising their professional practice in general and, in particular, the conditions for choosing the relevant intervention to solve the client's problem.

The conditions for SWs' and GPs' professional practice

The results of our study show that SWs and GPs identify clients in different ways, which means, first, that they have different images of who is a client. Second, this difference is of great significance for how they perform their professional practice. More concretely, their different perceptions of who is a client also affect their way of obtaining information about the client's problem and how it is to be solved. Put differently, it is evident that the conditions for SWs' and GPs' professional practice are different in many fundamental respects.

Applicant and client

There are two striking differences in the SW's and the GP's work of deciding who is a client. One is that *applicant* and *client* do not need to be the same person for SWs. Deciding who is a client is thus a starting point for SWs. On the other hand, for GPs there is no such discrepancy between applicant and client, since the two normally coincide. In other words, who is to be regarded as a client seems to be a non-question for GPs. The second difference is that in their dealings with clients, SWs immediately *zoom out*, while GPs *zoom in*. For SWs, zooming out means that they view the client in a wide social context. The following quotations show that SWs acknowledge that both parents and children may be affected by problems in the family and that they may all be in need of help.

> "It is time to call both parents. Employment is very important for the family.... They are at home and it's not good. There will certainly be tension between them, which will in turn affect the children, since they feel the tension between the parents." (SW5)

> "Of course, although Sara is asking for a personal meeting, in that case I would ask both Sara and her husband to come because this is about both of them as responsible parents." (SW6)

GPs on the other hand, as one GP puts it in one of the following quotations, zoom in to focus on the medical problem, for which social relations are considered to play a marginal role.

> "I don't start talking to the client about his wife and family.... I usually focus on the client. Starting to talk about children, a time comes when the client himself starts to open up and explain." (GP4)

> "And write nothing about anyone else!" (GP5)

> "No, no, that is what I was going to say. One shouldn't do that. I cannot, even if I have both of them as clients, I cannot write in Adam's records that Sara said this." (GP6)

A basic condition for all professional work is to decide who one's client is in order to initiate an intervention process. This is self-evident for GPs, which means that they can be described as a *monoclient profession* since their intervention process normally revolves around a single client. It is therefore easier for them to follow their routine intervention process from diagnosis to proposals for appropriate treatment. In contrast, SW's intervention process is often affected by a perceived discrepancy between applicant and client and by the fact that it is common for several people to be seen as tentative clients in any one case. Therefore, unlike GPs, they need to organise their intervention process according to several tentative clients' problems and needs. Social work can therefore be described as a *multiclient profession* since several tentative clients may be involved in the intervention process. SWs may need to review relationships within the family or the wider family network and consider who has the main problem and who, other than the client, is affected by the problem. This means that problem formulation in social work becomes very complex, since it is often an outcome of a negotiation process to get the client or clients to comply with the intervention process. SWs may also need to prepare motivational measures when clients are reluctant to identify themselves with the problem that an authority or an anonymous source ascribes to them. Thus being a mono- or multiclient profession is significant for how that profession obtains and assesses information.

Information

The two professions considered here differ even in such a fundamental way as obtaining information, which is a basic prerequisite for almost all professional work. The evident differences in these professions' ways of obtaining necessary or relevant information show that the conditions for enacting their professional practice are different. More concretely, these professions' ways of working with information differ in two respects. The first difference consists of *which* information, how much information and information about whom other than the client needs to be collected. SWs need both *personal information*, for example, about individual's specific problems, interests and needs, and *social information*, such as family situation, employment and social networks, about several tentative clients. In comparison, GPs mainly obtain only *personal* and *medical* information about the individual client. The second difference is about *how* or from whom the information is to be obtained. Unlike GPs, who have a single client as the main source, SWs need to gather information from sources other than the client in question.

What information and about whom?

Given that SWs regard persons other than the applicant as tentative clients, they need to seek wide-ranging information about the person or persons who are ascribed, or ascribe to themselves, client status. As the following quotation demonstrates, they need to gather information about the client's living conditions, social context and family situation, in order to assess how other tentative clients, such as children, are affected by the family circumstances.

> "I think we should bring in a good deal, their whole situation, to get a picture of what it looks like for these children and what the parents think about the children's situation.... And if we are to do what we want to do, we must also talk to the children." (SW1)

SWs have a legal obligation to gather wide-ranging and detailed information in order to make a comprehensive investigation. They must therefore actively seek information other than that obtained from the client. In contrast, GPs only have information about the individual client. The following quotation shows that GPs are primarily interested in the information that the client wishes to share.

> "We need to know what he wants us to know at first hand." (GP1)

Therefore, GPs do not need to seek other or more wide-ranging information about the client's social context and therefore take no account of second-hand information about the client. One reason, as the GP in the following excerpt reports, is that second-hand information probably has a negative effect the relationship between GP and client.

> "Exactly, information from the client's wife about his alcohol habits is absolutely not something to confront him with. There is no reason. That is just to question his honour. On the other hand, we can begin to talk about this in general terms." (GP1)

To the extent that GPs consider second-hand information, as the following quotation shows, they translate it into medical language, for example weaving second-hand information about the client's problematic drinking habits into a medical examination. The purpose is to validate or dismiss the information depending on whether it contains anything of substance about the client or is based on unfounded accusations to blacken the client. The most important information to GPs is therefore information about the body through anamnesis, existing medical records or new medical tests and examinations.

> "Obviously the wife's information about the client's alcohol habits will affect us. If there is a suspicion that this might be a great part of his problem, we must find a way of getting onto this track without revealing what the wife said, and this can be done by means of a hypertonic examination, so that this comes onto the table for discussion.' (GP2)

GPs are also clear about what information they do not wish to have. This includes information about the client's psycho-social problems. According to GPs, this type of information is more relevant to other professions, such as psychologists and hospital SWs.

Information sources

There are two striking differences in the two professions' attitudes to information sources. The first is that SWs use more information sources, since they need to have information about several tentative clients. The second is that SWs need to obtain information not only *from* the client but also *about* the client. Information *about* the client is not always gleaned from their own active search. They may also be provided with information by anonymous sources or by authorities who, on their own initiative, share with the SWs their concerns about children in disadvantaged family environments.

Information *about* the client gathered on the SWs' initiative is a consequence of their impression that the client is either providing fragmentary information or is intentionally withholding certain information. As the following quotations show, they need to request information *from* sources that have knowledge of the client and his or her family situation in order to make a thorough investigation, to compensate for fragmentary information from the client or to validate or reject biased information.

> "We obtain information from the school and preschool." (SW2)

> "We can obtain more information about the child's situation from the school by means of an assessment interview." (SW3)

SWs also need to consider second-hand information that comes via a formal report from an authority or an anonymous source. One of the SWs in our study explains how information in an anonymous report expressing concern about a child should be considered.

> "The information in this anonymous report focuses on concern for the child. Sometimes anonymous calls smear parents, but not in this case; this is genuine concern for the child, I think." (SW1)

Having many information sources naturally means that SWs have to make difficult decisions about the reliability of sources and the validity of the information. As this SW puts it, information *about* the client, obtained *from* an authority such as a school, is seen as more reliable than information *from* the client or *about* the client from an anonymous source.

> "Because we often also think that if the school or preschool do not report, they see the child five days a week, so we

> have quite a lot of confidence in the school or preschool, I would say. They have an obligation to report, so if things are this bad, then they should contact us." (SW1)

In comparison, GPs seldom face such a situation, since in their case the applicant, client and information source are normally the same person. This means that they regard the client as their main source of information, which makes it easier for them to make an assessment about the reliability of the information and its source. Seeking information about the client from another source, as the following quotation shows, is thus an unthinkable scenario for GPs.

> "This is a bit of a balancing act. It is only possible to use information that I have received in the discussion with Adam. We can only use the information in the discussion.... This moment is a bit delicate." (GP3)

To the extent that GPs need to obtain information *about* the client when they suspect that the client is withholding important information or providing inadequate information for some other reason, they seek physical evidence or refer to the information in the client's medical records. Physical evidence is gained by means of medical examinations and tests. This means that such physical evidence is 'encrypted' for the client, but not for the GP. The body is considered as an important information source that can be used to make the right diagnosis, but also to validate or reject the information that the GP receives from the client.

To summarise the discussion about information and information sources it is plausible to say that SWs handle a great deal of multifaceted and often conflicting information about several tentative clients. They therefore need to make difficult assessments about the validity of the information gathered and the importance and reliability of information sources, since confidence in, and the credibility of, the information source is a key aspect in the enactment of their professional practice. In contrast, confidence is normally built into GPs' relations with clients, since they generally have voluntary clients as the main source of information. Confidence, in combination with the fact that they have no legal obligation to obtain other information *about* the client, means that they have no need to devote a considerable part of the intervention process to assessing the information's reliability and winning the client's confidence.

Problems and problem solving

With the differences between SWs and GPs discussed in the previous section, it is hardly surprising that these professions also have different conceptions of problems and problem solving. The primary difference is that, compared with GPs, SWs often relate to the existence of parallel problems and solutions since they see many people as tentative clients. Because of this, SWs may find themselves in situations where efforts directed towards one client, for example, a child in a child protection case, can be perceived as having negative consequences for another client, such as a parent.

Put differently, SWs must make assessments of complex problem scenarios. They may direct efforts *to* parents, to help them improve their ability to provide care and thereby change or improve the child's situation. Efforts may also be directed *against* parents when, in addition to demonstrating deficient care capacity, they are unwilling to change or improve the child's situation. SWs can direct intervention *against* parents when they consider that certain serious problems, such as lack of parental ability, are not only the client's problem but also a social problem. In such cases, as the following quotation illustrates, they have responsibility or a legal obligation to handle the problem even if the measures to protect the child are directed *against* the parents.

> "The child is very important to me here. I have a responsibility towards him. I also think of other matters, but the child must have warm togs and I cannot trust such parents, so I call them and say to them: 'You receive monetary benefit; buy clothes for the child with the money and send the receipt to me so that I can be sure he has clothes.'" (SW4)

> "As a person in authority, I am responsible for the whole family." (SW6)

> "Mum and dad are away. Poor kids! This is completely crazy. They are not allowed to do this. Child protection must get involved immediately. I would think they would take the child into immediate custody." (SW7)

In comparison, GPs seldom find themselves in such situations. For them it is self-evident that, on the basis of the client's anamnesis, they must formulate a problem, investigate its causes and propose appropriate solutions to the problem. It is also self-evident to them that measures must be directed *towards* the client and nobody else and definitely not *against* the client unless there are specific reasons for doing so. It is also self-evident to them that it is the client who owns the problem, that their primary task is to solve the client's medical problems and that the client's psycho-social problems must be resolved by other professions. The following excerpts show how GPs feel that it is not their job to take over the client's problem and intervene in the client's life *against* his or her will.

> "Medical centre has good support from a hospital social worker and a psychologist and when cases such as this arise, which are family problems, I try to motivate them to turn to these if help is needed at home." (GP2)

> "This is actually not my problem. I should be careful to not make this my problem." (GP1)

The issue that who is to be viewed as a client is not self-evident for SWs means that they may find themselves in moral and legal dilemmas. Moral dilemmas arise when SWs get involved in situations where their legal obligations require them to intervene against the will of parents in order to protect a child. Such measures could on the one hand upset the parents' confidence in SWs. On the other hand, if SWs comply with the parents, they risk abandoning their legal obligations. Having several tentative clients in any one case also creates practical difficulties, since they must plan and coordinate different measures directed *to* or *against* clients with different interests. The GP's intervention process, in contrast, is focused on individual clients. In spite of the fact that a client may have a complex or comorbid problem, the GPs seldom find themselves with moral or legal dilemmas of the type that affect SWs. For GPs it is usually self-evident that the client owns the problem and that nobody else should be the subject of medical interventions. If they find indicators of the existence of parallel problems, for example if the client's psycho-social problems are thought to affect others, it is also self-evident to them that these must be handled by other professionals. It is thus plausible to say that the conditions for the professional practice of the two professions differ at the most basic level.

Theoretical and organisational implications of variations in the content of professional practice

This chapter has shown that SWs and GPs work systematically and rationally in their intervention processes insofar as they make a diagnosis, reasoning about clients and clients' problems, and propose appropriate treatments to solve the problems. It also shows that there is variation in the content of their intervention processes. Knowledge about these differences may have theoretical, political and organisational implications that can be considered when comparing and developing professions and making their practice evidence-based.

The first theoretical implication is that an understanding of different professions' intervention processes needs to be adapted according to the specific conditions for the enactment of their professional practice. In existing theories about professions' intervention processes (Hasenfeld, 1983; Abbott, 1988) this is normally described as a rational and linear process consisting of diagnosis, inference and treatment (DIT). This model is considered to reflect all professions' intervention processes. As Figure 15.1 illustrates, this model is more representative of the GP's intervention process, since this usually follows a linear and rational logic. This is partly due to the fact that, GPs, as a monoclient profession, often diagnose and treat a single client. GPs' narrow mandate in Sweden does not permit them, other than in exceptional cases such as the risk of infectious disease, to treat several clients (a whole family, for example) or make coercive interventions in clients' lives (Lipsky, 2010).

Moreover, the DIT model does not reflect all aspects of SWs' practice in Swedish personal social services since SWs, as a multiclient profession, have a wide and extended mandate that involves both care and coercion and allows them to intervene at both the personal and system level (Vindegg, 2009; Levin, 2013). Unlike GPs, whose mandate leaves little room for changing aspects other than the client's biophysical condition (Hasenfeld, 1983), the SW's mandate includes changing the client's social, economic, cognitive and affective condition. Thus a considerable limitation of the DIT model is not that it is unsuited to the SW's practice but rather that the SW's intervention process, as Figure 15.1 illustrates, can be best illustrated as a genealogical or family tree rather than a straight line. This is because the SW's mandate involves putting the client into a wider social context and investigating who else, other than the applicant or client, is affected by a problem and thereby needs help or protection.

Figure 15.1: Social workers' and GPs' intervention processes

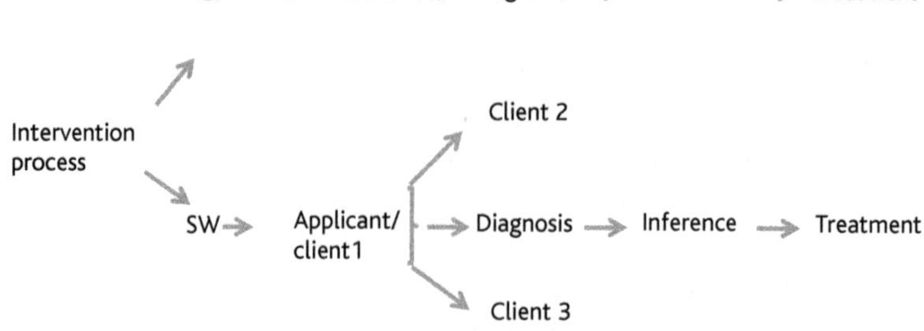

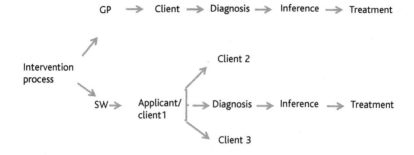

When it comes to implications for policymakers and organisational leaders, the differences illustrated by this chapter may be of significance in discussions about how to make the practice of non-medical professions evidence-based. One central aspect of the model for evidence-based practice is that professionals, in addition to best research evidence and clinical expertise, should also consider clients' preferences and values. Earlier research shows that even GPs as a monoclient profession can also have difficulties in using best evidence when the client refuses evidence-based measures (Rexvid et al, 2012). For a multiclient profession such as SWs, it can be even more difficult to consider the client's expectations and preferences since they often have several tentative clients, many of them involuntary, who have different problems and needs and conflicting interests. Moreover, SWs in Sweden have a legal obligation to use coercive interventions in clients' lives in specific cases. Such intervention occurs not on the basis of the client's preferences and expectations but rather on the basis of society's basic norms for protecting the client or others from the client's destructive behaviour or way of life. But this is not to say that coercive intervention does not occur with reference to best evidence of what is in the interests of the client or of society. This means that reforming, developing and standardising non-medical professions, which are expected to follow the principles that underpin evidence-based medicine, must occur on the basis of their specific conditions, since there is an obvious risk that 'one size fits nobody'. Different professions cannot be developed and subjected to evidence basing in exactly the same way, given that they have different mandates, are mono- or multiclient professions and have different intervention technologies. This political and organisational implication is linked to the second theoretical implication.

The second theoretical implication is that the differences that the chapter puts forward raise the question of whether it is reasonable or fruitful to hold up the medical profession as a role model for other welfare professions when there are fundamental differences in their enactment of professional practice. An obvious risk of regarding medical practice as the yardstick when comparing professions is that the characteristics of non-medical professions can be seen as deviations from the medical norm. A more fruitful comparative approach would be to regard the characteristics of non-medical professions as an important entrance into a nuanced understanding of their specific conditions for the enactment of their professional practice. It is thus central to the comparison of professions, in addition to considering scientific knowledge, legitimation, length of academic education, remuneration system and status, to take into account such factors as the content and range of different professions' mandates, whether they are mono- or multiclient professions and whatever technologies they have at their disposal. Otherwise the comparison risks becoming normative, which in turn recreates stereotypes and hierarchical patterns of occupational groups as professions and non-professions.

Note

1 The study is part of a larger research project entitled 'How do SWs and GPs use knowledge in practice', funded by the Swedish Research Council for Health, Working Life and Welfare.

References

Abbott, A. (1988) *The system of professions. An essay on the division of expert labor*, Chicago, IL: University of Chicago Press.

Brante, T. (2014) *Den professionella logiken: Hur vetenskap och praktik förenas i det moderna kunskapssamhället* [The professional logic: How science and practice unite in the modern knowledge society], Stockholm: Liber.

Brante, T., Johnsson, E., Olofsson, G. and Svensson, L.G. (2015) *Professionerna i kunskapssamhället: En jämförande studie av svenska professioner* [The professions in the knowledge society: A comparative study of Swedish professions], Stockholm: Liber.

Dellgran, P. (2015) 'Människobehandlande professioner' [Human service professions], in S. Johansson, P. Dellgran and S. Höjer (eds) *Människobehandlande organisationer. Villkor för ledning, styrning och professionellt välfärdsarbete* [Human service organisations. Conditions for management, control and welfare work], Stockholm: Natur and Kultur, pp 166-93.

Freidson, E. (1961) *Patients' views of medical practice*, New York, NY: Russell Sage Foundation.

Hasenfeld, Y. (1983) *Human service organizations*, Englewood Cliffs, NJ: Prentice-Hall.

Järvinen, M. (2002) 'Mötet mellan klient och system: om forskning i socialt arbete' [The encounter between client and system: on research in social work], *Dansk Sociologi*, 13(2): 73-84.

Järvinen, M. and Mik-Meyer, N. (eds) (2003) *At skabe en klient: Institutionelle identiteter i socialt arbejde* [Constructing a client: Institutional identities in social work], København: Hans Reitzel.

Johnson, T.J. (1972) *Professions and power*, London: Macmillan.

Levin, C. (2013) 'Socialt arbete som moralisk praktik'[Social work as moral practice], in S. Linde and K. Svensson (eds) *Förändringens entreprenörer och tröghetens agenter: Människobehandlande organisationer ur ett nyinstitutionellt perspektiv* [The entrepreneurs of change and the agents of interia: Human service organisations from a new institutional perspective] (1st edn), Stockholm: Liber, pp 25-41.

Lipsky, M. (2010) *Street-level bureaucracy: dilemmas of the individual in public services*, (30th anniversary expanded edn) New York, NY: Russell Sage Foundation.

Molander, A. and Terum, L. I. (2010) 'Profesjonsstudier – en introduksjon' [Studies in professions – an introduction], in A. Molander and L.I. Terum (eds) *Profesjonsstudier* [Studies in professions], Oslo: Universitetsforlaget, pp 13-27.

Mosesson, M. (2000) 'Intervention', in V. Denvall and T. Jacobson (eds) *Var- dagsbegrepp i socialt arbete. Ideologi, teori och praktik* [Everyday concepts in social work. Ideology, theory and practice], Stockholm: Norstedts Juridik, pp 223-40.

Rexvid, D., Blom, B., Evertsson, L. and Forssén, A. (2012) 'Risk reduction technologies in general practice and social work', *Professions and Professionalism*, 2(2): 1-18.

Salonen, T. (2000) 'Klient' [Client], in I V. Denvall & T. Jacobson (eds) *Vardagsbegrepp i socialt arbete. Ideologi, teori och praktik* [Everyday concepts in social work. Ideology, theory and practice], Stockholm: Norstedts Juridik.

Svensson, L.G. (2010) 'Profesjon og organisasjon' [Profession and organisation], in A. Molander and L.I. Terum (eds) *Profesjonsstudier* [Studies in professions], Oslo: Universitetsforlaget, pp 130-43.

Vindegg, J. (2009) 'Evidensbasert socialt arbeid' [Evidence-based social work], in H. Grimen and L.I. Terum (eds) *Evidensbasert profesjonutøvelse* [Evidence-based professional work], Oslo: Abstrakt forlag, pp 63-85.

SIXTEEN

Activation work as professional practice: complexities and professional boundaries at the street level of employment policy implementation

Urban Nothdurfter and Søren Peter Olesen

Introduction

Recent developments in European social and employment policy represent fluid and contradictory conditions and trends for street-level practice in employment-related services. This chapter addresses these issues in three different European contexts: Italy, Austria and Denmark. The chapter is based mainly on two separate studies, one covering street-level work in the employment services in Vienna and Milan, the other covering a variety of Danish municipal jobcentres. The aim of the chapter is to discuss the challenges for street-level, employment-oriented work, including the question of the relevance of professional knowledge and practice, with reference to similarities and differences between the three European contexts mentioned. The chapter is theoretically framed by a street-level bureaucracy perspective (Lipsky, 2010), highlighting the important role of street-level workers whose interactions and uses of discretion on the front line of employment-related services make a significant contribution to employment policy implementation.

Developments in European social and employment policy represent a shift from a 'one size fits all' welfare state towards more decentred and individualised forms of welfare state intervention (Barbier and Ludwig-Mayerhofer, 2004; Heidenreich and Aurich Beerheide, 2014). In this context, factors related to the operational side of policy, including front-line practice in employment-related services, are increasingly taken into account (Brodkin and Marston, 2013). The day-to-day operation of the activating welfare state strongly relies on the changed interaction at the front line of services (Meyers et al, 1998; McDonald and Marston, 2005) and the call for tailormade services implies a stronger and more discretionary role for front-line practitioners (van Berkel et al, 2010). However, complexities and professional boundaries in the street-level implementation of employment policy still need to be better explored in order to gain a deeper understanding of how the ambiguities and contradictions of activation eventually unfold in practice and of how practitioners move between the de-professionalised, administrative routines on the one hand and the demands of professional practice on the other.

These questions are even more topical as professional work in public welfare services is generally challenged (Noordegraaf and Steijn, 2013). Professions once perceived as agents in the establishment and further development of the welfare state have been increasingly under pressure and their knowledge base represents a challenge to policy developments. At the same time, some contributions have pointed out a shift from a bureaucratic towards a more professional approach of front-line work in public services combined with the introduction of performance-oriented styles of management (Noordegraaf, 2007; van Berkel et al, 2010). However, in the field of employment policy, this demand for professionalism has to be observed carefully as it is still rather uncertain what professional work should mean in this ambiguous domain. This uncertainty is not least reflected by different ideas and situations regarding the involvement of professionals like social workers with their knowledge and professional ethics in this context (Kjørstad, 2005; van Berkel and van der Aa, 2012).

Different policy frameworks have a strong influence on front-line practice and, thus, also on the content and range of practitioners' agency, particularly when it comes to clients who present additional difficulties and do not 'fit' into the prevailing activation agenda of quick labour market integration (Rice, 2015). In this sense, a comparative view helps to address more specifically the central questions regarding professional demands and challenges in employment efforts. What is the specific character of the street-level implementation of employment policy or 'activation work' in different contexts? Is it professional work or rather a matter of de-professionalised, administrative routines? Does this type of work represent a separate form of professional knowledge and ethics?

The Italian case

Italian labour market policy has traditionally been characterised by strong insider protection. Against this background, the activation paradigm entered the Italian political agenda rather hesitantly and active policies have been developed for a long time in a rather half-hearted and fragmented way (Calza Bini and Lucciarini, 2013). While different labour market reforms from the second half of the 1990s were aimed mainly at the flexibilisation of the labour market (Sacchi and Vesan, 2015), governance reforms pointed to a multi-level and non-hierarchical governance model promoting processes of decentralisation and marketisation of employment-related services (Graziano and Raué, 2011). As these reform attempts have been implemented very differently on the sub-national level, a general characterisation of Italy is, however, difficult and the governance of activation eventually depends on the policies and institutional capabilities of the regions (and even provinces) (Ambra et al, 2013).

Since 2012, new labour market reforms have extended social protection and further emphasised the need for improving national strategies for the promotion of active policies, not least through the foundation of a national employment agency (Zilio Grandi and Biasi, 2016).

Italian labour market policy is, however, still characterised by a highly fragmented situation with different landscapes of activation. Furthermore, there is a lack of institutional coordination, not only between labour market and social policies generally, but even between the administration of unemployment benefits and the delivery of employment-related services. Moreover, social protection policies continue to be weak and additional social and care services are lacking.

The Province of Milan has reformed its public employment services, setting up special agencies for training, guidance and work (*Agenzie per la formazione, l'orientamento e il lavoro*, or AFOL) that cover the whole metropolitan area of Milan. They were founded with the idea of a general relaunch and integration of public employment, orientation and training services. In the city of Milan, services are provided by the AFOL Milano, set up as an umbrella organisation that has incorporated different formerly separated services, such as the public employment service and career guidance and vocational training centres. AFOL Milano offers a spectrum of employment-related services to both citizens and employers.

The specific character of street-level implementation of employment policy in Milan

Despite the intent of better integration, in practice the tasks of the classical employment-related bureaucracy continue to be carried out within different service units and by different front-line staff.

As exploratory research on front-line identities and practice representations of practitioners engaged in the provision of employment-related services[1] has shown, this divide notably determines the specific character of front-line practice (Nothdurfter, 2014, 2016). As the tasks of the employment-related bureaucracy are hardly linked with the provision of services, practitioners are less exposed to the dilemmas of activation. In fact, practitioners involved in the provision of services can concentrate on enabling aspects as the clients they work with engage with them primarily on a voluntary basis, and thus tend to have better chances from the outset.

In their practice representations, street-level workers in Milan emphasise the notions of individualised help and support without perceiving them as being at odds with their given mandate. The latter is, in fact, not defined as ending unemployment as soon as possible but as orienting and supporting people in their autonomous jobseeking and labour market integration process. Against this background, the importance of understanding jobseekers' individual situations is depicted as the main starting point for a professional intervention and the notion of providing individualised support is represented as the specific character of this type of work, with all the difficulties and gratifications of a professional activity based on a helping relationship.

Accordingly, practitioners' interpretations of the notion of activation work reflect its positive aspects and its enabling dimension. However, at the same time practitioners seem to miss somehow its demanding side, stating that their efforts of activating people are not equally matched by clear activity requirements and by making benefit receipt conditional (which is, however, depicted as the job of 'others'). In this regard, practitioners in Milan seem to be quite ambivalent. While they point out the importance of working on a non-compulsory basis and of improving people's autonomy when they speak about their own job, they seem to embrace ambiguities and contradictory conditions and trends in employment policy in a rather uncritical way.

Practitioners in Milan come from different educational and professional backgrounds, with some of them having a specific qualification for occupational orientation and counselling. However, the field of street-level implementation of employment policy does not involve professional social workers and a discussion about whether a social work approach could be relevant in this type of work seems not to be under way.

To sum up, the Italian case is a latecomer in activation with fragmented, local active labour market policy regimes that lack coordination between employment-related and social policies and services. As the case of public employment services in Milan shows, the street-level implementation of employment policy is still characterised by the lack of integration in tasks of registration, control and placement (considered as mere bureaucratic work) and support services such as orientation and counselling. This means that in practice contradictory policy trends come less to the fore and practitioners involved in providing support services continue to have ample space for autonomous agency.

Furthermore, this kind of street-level work is represented as a challenging professional activity, which requires professional attitudes and skills. However, its specific character seems to be rather limited within an individually oriented counselling paradigm (and so is the relevant knowledge base) and the support services offered are not equalled by effective matching or placement services and training schemes. There is a professional framing of employment-related front-line work (or rather of certain front-line activities) on the one hand, while on the other a lack of integrated support towards employment persists. Practice representations are framed within the realm of a classical professional activity without taking into account contradictory aspects of employment policy.

The Austrian case

Since the 1990s, Austria has reoriented its labour market policies, combining social security provisions with extended labour market flexibility and giving priority to so-called active measures over passive unemployment benefit receipt (Stelzer-Orthofer, 2011). The most important reform in this context was introduced in 1994, providing a new legal framework regarding both the normative and the organisational dimension of employment policy. With this reform, the Austrian public employment service was formally separated from the ministry of labour and a semi-autonomous, tripartite public employment service agency (Arbeitsmarktservice, or AMS) was established. The reform also marked an increase in the relevance of activation strategies and early interventions in order to achieve quick and sustainable labour market integration of jobseekers.

The establishment of the AMS aimed to transform the public employment service from a bureaucratic employment office into a comprehensive service provider, pursuing the goals of abandoning the state monopoly in placement, decentralising decision-making processes and increasing both the flexibility in regional deployment of resources and the better involvement of social partners. This transformation has been marked also by the introduction of New Public Management strategies with a strong emphasis on management by objectives techniques (BMASK, 2013).

The cooperation between the public employment service and local welfare offices has increased substantially, especially with the introduction of a new minimum income scheme in 2010. Although Austria has not merged public employment and local welfare services, social assistance recipients capable of working have to register at the AMS and participate in activation measures. Their performance and compliance is reported to local welfare offices, which decide on the possible curtailing of minimum income benefits (Leibetseder et al, 2015).

The specific character of street-level implementation of employment policy in Vienna

The Austrian context combines a responsibility-based understanding of unemployment and an emphasis on quick labour market integration (Atzmüller, 2009) with strong investment in employment-related services (BMASK, 2013). Employment policy has a strong contractualistic trait based on individual activation agreements.

The organisational structure of the AMS in the city of Vienna comprises a federal state office for Vienna, 12 local branch offices located around the city and a specialised office for young jobseekers aged up to 21 years. Each branch office is organised in different service units ('zones') that offer information, registration for placement claims and benefit receipt and, within the so-called counselling zone, intensive guidance and assistance for jobseekers and benefit recipients.

Exploring the challenges for practitioners working in the counselling zone of the AMS offices in Vienna has shown that the clearer approach to activation in Austrian employment policy has substantial consequences for front-line practice (Nothdurfter, 2014, 2016). Demanding and enabling aspects of employment policy have to be held together and practitioners have a crucial role in combining and balancing them in individual situations. This is not that evident at first sight as practitioners have to follow standardised procedures, rules and legal provisions and are accountable to strict managerial control with particular attention on how many of the enrolled clients take up a job or pass into long-term unemployment.

However, beneath this regulative framework, practitioners dispose of discretional spaces. This is not surprising as they have to cope with the classical dilemmas of street-level bureaucracies. The interesting question is, though, how the use of discretion occurs against the background of how front-line work is conceptualised and interpreted in the activation context. On the one hand, front-line work is first and foremost understood, even in the counselling zone, as the application of unemployment insurance provisions and as such is still designed as a rather administrative activity. This understanding is reflected also by formal qualification requirements. Practitioners are not required to hold a professional qualification (even though some of the interviewed practitioners come from a social work or similar background) but are qualified in special in-house training areas. On the other hand, practitioners' accounts show that the street-level implementation of employment policy requires overcoming a mere bureaucratic understanding of front-line work and applying more nuanced approaches that involve different sources of knowledge as well as ethical considerations.

These accounts reflect the dilemmas of an activity that continues to be designed as a predominantly administrative one in the face of increasing 'professional' challenges. Some practitioners seem to assume a stronger caring attitude and argue for taking individual difficulties more into account. Others assume a more bureaucratic attitude, pointing out that they cannot help but just follow the rules, while still others argue mainly in favour of the bigger policy goal of bringing people out of benefit receipt and into work as quickly as possible. Furthermore, practitioners interpret the notion of activation in very different ways, depending on different target groups and situations. In this sense, the street-level implementation of employment policy constitutes a rather ambiguous field of practice in which administrative routines and complex challenges clash and in which the ways practitioners understand their job and assess their clients along the axes of employability and willingness result in different activation practices.

In interviews practitioners emphasise the dimension of individualised help and support, especially with regard to those target groups that do not fit well into the agenda of quick labour market integration. They report being increasingly confronted with people who have multiple difficulties and for whom unemployment is only one and often even not the most pressing problem. In these cases, practitioners have to recognise that labour market integration or training cannot constitute primary goals and are often even not realistic, at least in the short term. Practitioners emphasise the importance of a 'human' approach to such situations, which respects people's difficulties and avoids demanding the impossible. However, this attitude is represented rather in terms of a personal concern and endeavour than a professional responsibility.

Challenges encountered in practice risk falling back and being dealt with on a rather personal level by the individual practitioner. This marginalisation of professional challenges to an individualistic and personal rather than professional sphere is even more remarkable as some practitioners are, at the same time, quite explicit about the structural nature of the conflicts they have to face. One aspect pointed out in this context concerns the nature of the public employment service itself. It is represented as a user-oriented service provider while overseeing sovereign public functions, including control and sanctions. In this sense, the public employment service itself is perceived as a rather ambiguous entity whose double-faced nature is broken down to practice and, eventually, unfolds in interactions with service users, especially those who are most disadvantaged in terms of their employability.

The Austrian case shows that a stronger orientation towards activation in employment and social policy has not been matched by a consistent professionalisation project of street-level work in the public employment service. The street-level implementation of employment policy constitutes a highly individualised (and at least potentially also arbitrary) project where clients run the risk of being greatly at the mercy of those they encounter and front-line practitioners themselves are exposed to a precarious self-reliance in coping with their difficult job.

The Danish case

Denmark is traditionally characterised by a flexible labour market with low insider protection and to a large extent a universalistic social security system. Combined with social policy changes regarding cash benefit recipients, a major labour market reform in 1994 covering the insured unemployed marked a general and gradual shift from welfare to workfare during the 1990s (Torfing, 2004). A further reform came in 2002, with the initiative '*Flere i arbejde*' or 'More people into jobs', marking a shift from a 'human capital' to a 'work first' strategy and intensified New Public Management governance. Social policy is turned into *employment policy*, implying that social welfare clients in principle are treated like other unemployed people and today are categorised according to their readiness either for employment or participation in activation work.

One of the main steps in this process is the merging of the state employment services and the municipal social welfare and employment offices into *municipal jobcentres* in 2009. The Danish jobcentre reform follows a major administrative reform of local government in 2007, reducing the number of municipalities from 279 to 98. The reform implies decentralisation. At the same time, intensified governance measures set up clear limits for local government. The way jobcentres are organised, however, varies considerably. As a consequence, employment issues for insured as well as uninsured unemployed people are managed by municipal jobcentres (Bredgaard et al, 2011).

Danish Labour market and social policy is a case of *flexicurity*, referring to a comparatively high level of both flexibility and social security, including, as an important element, an emphasis on active policy measures, expenditures being high on both security and active measures (Bredgaard et al, 2011). Although the financial crisis silenced some of the optimism surrounding flexicurity, it is still functioning (Bredgaard and Kongshøj Madsen, 2015)

During the period 2011-15 parts of the 'work first' strategy were rolled back (and again reintroduced in 2015), while other parts intensified. Administrative changes including rehabilitation teams, coordinating casework and individual treatment programmes, focusing on resources rather than problems, scrutinised the importance of the organisation and the knowledge base at the street level in order to, among other things, prevent increasing numbers on social pension schemes. A cash benefit reform in 2014 emphasised the obligation on benefit recipients under the age of 30 to take work or start education. Despite the focus on the complexities of problems among cash benefit recipients, governance measures, including control and sanctioning, are still being scrutinised.

Such policy changes over time deeply influence street-level activities and demands on staff qualifications. Although the overall picture represents an unequivocal turn to active policies, there is constant space for discretion in activation work. Furthermore, working with vulnerable cash benefit recipients and people on sick leave demands *professionalism* (Baadsgaard et al, 2014a, 2014b, 2014c).

The specific character of street-level implementation of employment policy

A major Danish study[2] shows differences and disagreements across jobcentres as well as internally, for instance between management and street-level workers. Emphasis on professional qualifications and competences, further, is more prominent among street-level workers than among managers and less prominent among cash benefit than sick leave recipients. Employment orientation and an emphasis on self-support as the basic principle is widespread, but the strategies vary considerably among the jobcentres. Correspondingly, approaches and judgements regarding the demand for professional competences and the relevance of different professional groups vary significantly. And among the jobcentres selected for in-depth analysis, even if they share a common rationale generally emphasising activation and employment, four different strategies appear: *job placement; job clarification; clarification of the future support needs of the citizen*; and, finally, *ongoing activation, control and sanctions* (Baadsgaard et al, 2014c, emphasis added).

Across the shared rationale and strategic differences between the jobcentres, dilemmas, scepticism and reservations appear among some of the street-level workers. Street-level workers report autonomy and discretion, albeit at a reduced level due to regulation and standardisation, and they experience a discrepancy between employment policy goals, including the line or strategy of the jobcentre, and the needs, characteristics and competences of the client group. Street-level workers experience ethical dilemmas as a result of bureaucratic rules and rigid procedures, and problematise the policy emphasis on employment and activation, especially when talking about vulnerable groups (Baadsgaard et al, 2014b).

Jobcentre managers, on the contrary, argue along different lines and define their role as follows:

- To 'turn' people already at the jobcentre entrance and motivate them to move 'back to work', with a focus on 'administration of activation and control measures'. In this context, administrative and organisational competences are demanded and there is no need for professionals.
- To clarify the needs of unemployed cash benefit and sick leave recipients in terms of social diagnosis, treatment and helping people to find solutions to social problems. In this context, there is a clear need for professional social workers.
- To help people back to work in terms of finding practice placements, training and education opportunities or job openings as well as

> helping people to manage their life situation while in activation and employment. In this context, there is a need for an employment-oriented professional practice. Professionals will, however, be able to give activation, work and education priority (Baadsgaard et al, 2014b).

A survey gives further insight into this, showing that 76% of jobcentre staff have a professional or academic education, and more than 40% of staff at Danish jobcentres are trained social workers (Baadsgaard et al, 2014a). What street-level workers find professionally relevant and important are a holistic approach to the citizen, conversational and guidance skills, and knowledge of public law and employment policy rules and measures; knowledge about the labour market and educational opportunities, meanwhile, is less emphasised. The measures given highest priority among street-level workers are thorough and precise instructions and using the wishes and demands of the citizen as a starting point for the employment effort. In contrast reminding the street-level worker about the economic penalties they will incur should they fail to attend regular meetings at the jobcentre, or actively apply for work, are considered less important (Baadsgaard et al, 2014a).

In conclusion, what jobcentre staff tend to consider relevant is to a considerable degree in accordance with the central principles of social work, leading to a discussion of the relationship between social work and what is needed in street-level work at jobcentres. For some street-level workers, the dilemmas tend to overshadow the possibilities. Among some jobcentre managers, there is a parallel scepticism towards professional social workers, while others prefer professional social workers or street-level workers with comparable qualifications. So, from some perspectives social work does not appear as relevant for the implementation of employment policy, just as from a critical social work perspective, jobcentres might not offer relevant jobs for professional social workers (Baadsgaard et al, 2014c).

The discussion raised in the Danish study problematises both points of view. There is a tradition in Danish social work for rehabilitation (*revalidering*), for instance following an accident or severe health problems, which most of the time has been closely associated with the administration of welfare benefits and the aim of self-maintenance. So, it can be argued that it is not incompatible with social work ethics, values and skills to work with efforts that aim at employment and self-support (Olesen, 2011). And, finally, as regards the challenges and demands associated with work at the jobcentres, social work qualifications meet these to a considerable extent (Baadsgaard et al, 2014c).

Conclusion

The three cases confirm that emphasis on activation makes street-level practice and individualised service provision an increasingly important policy arena. Standardisation, control and sanctions stand out. Where activation policies strongly link employment and social policy goals, street-level practice is faced with complex challenges and contradictory conditions. This is the case especially when it comes to work with more vulnerable groups. Street-level workers often perceive a strong discrepancy between policy emphasis and the characteristics of different client groups, and experience challenging ethical dilemmas in responding to both employment goals and peoples' needs. Moving across the three examples, this appears to be the case even more when active measures are emphasised and particularly, as in the Danish case, when employment and social welfare services are merged.

At the same time, the contours of street-level implementation of employment-oriented policies or 'activation work' as a professional practice are still rather unclear. These activities involve a strong share of administrative work with de-professionalised and standardised bureaucratic routines and procedures. At the same time, there seems to be considerably high expectations as regards the effects of activation efforts and a growing need and awareness for responses aimed at the solution of social problems that obstruct ways back to employment. Furthermore, activation work also involves a disciplinary character hardly compatible with professional knowledge and ethics. In short, activation work appears as a set of Janus-faced practices that involve critical elements and both de-professionalised routines and rising demands of professionalism. Street-level work appears as challenging, particularly if participation in work activities is seen as part of the solution to social problems rather than the final goal. The professionalisation of activation work, however, is still in its infancy.

In Milan, the fragmented approach to employment and activation policies allows for the professional framing of some aspects of job counselling, while other aspects of the street-level implementation of employment policy continue to be carried out within a system of traditional employment bureaucracy.

In Vienna, practitioners are much more exposed to the dilemmas of activation. However, front-line work continues to be conceptualised and designed as an administrative activity and practitioners have few possibilities to deal with the complex challenges of their job within the realm of a professional scope. Challenges redound on a rather personal sphere of practitioners' sensibility and responsiveness. Clients depend heavily on practitioners' responses and practitioners themselves are exposed to precarious self-reliance.

In the Danish context, as a result of merging the employment service with social welfare, activation work is to a large extent carried out by a professional group, mostly trained social workers, coming from the social welfare offices. The demand for professionalism in activation work, however, is disputed. Some jobcentre managers emphasise the administrative character of activation work, just as some professionals are sceptical about whether there is any room left for professional methods, values and ethics. Nonetheless, within the Danish debate there is an emphasis on the need for a deeper and more concrete knowledge about employment and education opportunities as well as a more holistic approach to citizens' situations and a professional focus on the treatment of problems related to unemployment.

Against this background, we argue that a more social work-oriented approach may contribute to the debate on street-level implementation of employment policy. Current policy developments imply challenges for, as well as from such, an approach concerning the seemingly ubiquitous emphasis on employment, especially regarding people with problems in addition to unemployment. In other fields, as well, professional social work has developed out of this core dilemma: to be linked to official policy goals, but to strive, at the same time, for autonomy based on a separate form of professional knowledge and ethics committed to the needs expressed by those who constitute the target groups of social policy. Add to this a demand for detailed knowledge about opportunities as well as limitations according to law, about physical and mental health problems and the health system, about local labour market relations and education opportunities, and about negotiation and relational competences. It is likely that all this is needed for the professionalisation of activation work. Not an 'either-or' solution but an 'as-well-as' approach, able to recapture a balance between employment-oriented goals and solutions to complex social problems, based on ethical standards and opened up for negotiation with the citizens concerned.

Notes

1 The paragraphs on the Italian and the Austrian case empirically draw on an explorative case study undertaken on the front line of public employment services in the cities of Milan and Vienna between November 2011 and March 2012. The research aimed at studying challenges, interpretations and reactions as experienced and depicted by front-line practitioners. Data was collected by qualitative interviews combining a vignette technique with flexible interview guidelines in order to give practitioners space for their narrative accounts (Nothdurfter, 2014, 2016).

[2] The analysis of the Danish case is based on an overall mixed-method study of the work of jobcentres concerning employment measures, particularly regarding vulnerable cash benefit recipients and people on sick leave (Baadsgaard et al, 2014a, 2014b, 2014c.)

References

Ambra, M.C., Cortese, C. and Pirone, F. (2013) 'Geografie di attivazione: regolazione e governance fra scala regionale e variabilità locale' [Geography of activation: regulation and governance of regional and local scale variability], in Y. Kazepov and E. Barberis (eds) *Il welfare frammentato: Le articolazioni regionali delle politiche sociali italiane* [The fragmented welfare: Regional articulations of Italian social policies], Roma: Carocci, pp 89-109.

Atzmüller, R. (2009) 'Aktivierung statt Vollbeschäftigung. Die Entwicklung der Arbeitsmarktpolitik in Österreich' [Activation instead of full employment. The development of labour market policy in Austria], in C. Hermann and R. Atzmüller (eds) *Die Dynamik des österreichischen Modells: Brüche und Kontinuitäten im Beschäftigungs- und Sozialsystem* [The dynamics of the Austrian model: Ruptures and continuities in the employment and social system], Berlin: Edition Sigma, pp 135-86.

Baadsgaard, K., Jørgensen, H., Nørup, I. and Olesen, S.P. (2014a) *Jobcentre og klemte kvalifikationer*, [Jobcentres and squeezed qualifications], Aalborg: Aalborg Universitetsforlag.

Baadsgaard, K., Jørgensen, H., Nørup, I. and Olesen, S.P. (2014b) *Den faglige praksis i jobcentrene*, [The professional practice in jobcentres], Aalborg: Aalborg Universitetsforlag.

Baadsgaard, K., Jørgensen, H., Nørup, I. and Olesen, S.P. (2014c) *Beskæftigelsesfaglighed-Mikroprocesser i jobcentrenes frontlinje og kvalificeringsbehov* [Employment-oriented professionalism – Micro-processes at the street-level of jobcentres and demands for qualifications], Aalborg: Aalborg Universitetsforlag.

Barbier, J.-C. and Ludwig-Mayerhofer, W. (2004) 'Introduction: the many worlds of activation', *European Societies*, 6(4): 423-36.

BMASK (Bundesministerium für Arbeit, Soziales und Konsumentenschutz) (ed) (2013) *Aktive Arbeitsmarktpolitik in Österreich 1994-2013* [Active labour market policies in Austria 1994-2013], Wien: BMASK.

Bredgaard, T., Jørgensen, H., Madsen, P.K. and Rasmussen, S. (2011) *Dansk arbejdsmarkedspolitik*, [Danish labour market policy], Copenhagen: Jurist- og Økonomforbundets Forlag.

Bredgaard, T. and Kongshøj Madsen, P. (eds) (2015) *Dansk flexicurity: Fleksibilitet og sikkerhed på arbejdsmarkedet*, [Danish flexicurity: Flexibility and security in the labour market], Copenhagen: Hans Reitzels Forlag.

Brodkin, E.Z. and Marston, G. (eds) (2013) *Work and the welfare state: Street-level organizations and workfare politics*, Copenhagen: DJØF Publishing.

Calza Bini, P. and Lucciarini, S. (2013) 'La disarticolazione delle politiche del lavoro tra spinte, quadro nazionale e impulsi locali' [The disarticulation of the labour policies between pressure of national framework and local impulses], in Y. Kazepov and E. Barberis (eds) *Il welfare frammentato: Le articolazioni regionali delle politiche sociali italiane* [The fragmented welfare: Regional articulations of Italian social policies], Roma: Carocci, pp 73-88.

Graziano, P.R. and Raué, A. (2011) 'The governance of activation policies in Italy: from centralized and hierarchical to a multi-level open system model', in R. van Berkel, W. de Graaf and T. Sirovatka (eds) *The governance of active welfare states in Europe*, Basingstoke: Palgrave Macmillan, pp 110-31.

Heidenreich, M. and Aurich Beerheide, P. (2014) 'European worlds of inclusive activation: the organisational challenges of coordinated service provision', *International Journal of Social Welfare*, 23: S6-S22.

Kjørstad, M. (2005) 'Between professional ethics and bureaucratic rationality: the challenging ethical position of social workers who are faced with implementing a workfare policy', *European Journal of Social Work*, 8(4): 381-98.

Leibetseder, B., Altreiter, C. and Leitgöb, H. (2015) 'The new means-tested minimum income in Austria: discretion and regulation in practice', *Journal of Poverty and Social Justice*, 23(1): 57-70.

Lipsky, M. (2010) [1980] *Street-level bureaucracy: Dilemmas of the individual in public services* (30th anniversary expanded edn), London: Russell Sage.

McDonald, C. and Marston, G. (2005) 'Workfare as welfare: governing unemployment in the advanced liberal state', *Critical Social Policy*, 25(3): 374-401.

Meyers, M.K., Glaser, B. and MacDonald, K. (1998) 'On the front lines of welfare delivery: are workers implementing policy reforms?', *Journal of Policy Analysis and Management*, 17(1): 1-22.

Noordegraaf, M. (2007) 'From "pure" to "hybrid" professionalism: present-day professionalism in ambiguous public domains', *Administration & Society*, 39(6): 761-85.

Noordegraaf, M. and Steijn, B. (eds) (2013) *Professionals under pressure: The reconfiguration of professional work in changing public services*, Amsterdam: Amsterdam University Press.

Nothdurfter, U. (2014) 'Getting the job done...!? (Professional) challenges on the frontline of public employment services in Vienna and Milan', PhD thesis, University of Trento.

Nothdurfter, U. (2016) 'The street-level delivery of activation policies: constraints and possibilities for a practice of citizenship', *European Journal of Social Work*, 19(3-4): 420-40.

Olesen, S.P. (2011) 'Helhedssyn nedefra – et bottom up-perspektiv på social arbejde' [Holism from below – a bottom-up perspective on social work], in M. Harder and M.A. Nissen (eds) *Helhedssyn i socialt arbejde* [Holism in social work], Copenhagen: Akademisk Forlag, pp 213-37.

Rice, D. (2015) *Building active welfare states: How policy shapes caseworker practice*, Amsterdam: Vrije University Press.

Sacchi, S. and Vesan, P. (2015) 'Employment policy: segmentation, deregulation and reforms in the Italian labour market' in U. Ascoli and E. Pavolini (eds) *The Italian welfare state in a European perspective: A comparative analysis*, Bristol: Policy Press, pp 71-99.

Stelzer-Orthofer, C. (2011) 'Mindestsicherung und Aktivierung – Strategien der österreichischen Arbeitsmarktpolitik' [Minimum benefit and activation – strategies of Austrian labour market policy] in C. Stelzer-Orthofer and J. Weidenholzer (eds) *Aktivierung und Mindestsicherung: Nationale und europäische Strategien gegen Armut und Arbeitslosigkeit* [Activation and minimum benefit: National and European policies against poverty and unemployment], Wien: Mandelbaum Verlag, pp 141-56.

Torfing, J. (2004) *Det stille sporskifte i velfærdsstaten. En diskursteoretisk beslutningsprocesanalyse* [The silent switch in the welfare state. A discourse theoretical analysis of the decision-making processes], Århus: Aarhus Universitetsforlag.

van Berkel, R. and van der Aa, P. (2012) 'Activation work: policy programme administration or professional service provision?', *Journal of Social Policy*, 41(3): 493-510.

van Berkel, R., van der Aa, P. and van Gestel, N. (2010) 'Professionals without a profession? Redesigning case management in Dutch local welfare agencies', *European Journal of Social Work*, 13(4): 447-63.

Zilio Grandi, G. and Biasi, M. (eds) (2016) *Commentario breve alla riforma "Jobs Act"* [Short commentary on the "Jobs Act" reform], Padova: Cedam.

SEVENTEEN

Social and caring professions in European welfare states: trends and challenges

Marek Perlinski, Björn Blom and Lars Evertsson

Introduction

This book consists of four sections that address different aspects that are important to European social and caring welfare professions: knowledge, reflection and identity in the social and caring welfare professions; control, regulation and management; collaboration, conflict and competition; and assessment, negotiation and decision making. In this final chapter, we concentrate on a number of key issues from the book's various contributions to see what we can learn from them. The expression that 'Prediction is very difficult, especially about the future' is usually attributed to the Danish physicist Niels Bohr. With this reservation in mind, we declare that we have tried to take a look into the 'crystal ball', by spotting trends and tendencies that simultaneously say something about the current situation and offer a hint about future developments.

In the prior chapters, researchers from different countries and academic disciplines have tackled a number of queries and issues that are of concern for understanding the situation of current European social and caring welfare professions. We do not suggest that these queries have been given definite answers or that every important aspect has been examined. We believe, however, that the various contributions offer new insights about current welfare professions and their practices in a number of European welfare states.

This chapter begins with a discussion regarding a theme that is emphasised in several of the book's contributions and thus appears particularly crucial. One of the strongest trends in the book is the central, and maybe increasingly important, role that individual welfare states have in relation to social and caring welfare professions. Several authors point to what is probably a new phenomenon, at least regarding its prevalence – namely, that we still lack the proper conceptual and theoretical frameworks for understanding. In other words, the state sometimes instantaneously creates entirely new professions alongside established professions, or creates entirely new organisational and administrative forms that suddenly abolish or change existing professional jurisdictions.

This discussion is followed by a section that concentrates on social and caring welfare professionals' identity, and how identities may be in a state of flux, as a result of different forms of state involvement. The chapter then addresses various struggles and conflicts between different professional groups in new organisational settings, as well as emerging conflicts between welfare professions and the state. This is followed by a section discussing whether knowledge is a tool for professionals, as we usually tend to think, or a means for controlling professionals in more or less subtle ways. The chapter ends with some concluding remarks.

The state gives, the state takes and the state alters the rules of the game

As researchers have noticed, the relationship between the welfare state and its social and caring welfare professions has changed. Closely related to the expansion of the welfare state was the development of welfare professionals. Welfare professions were intimately woven into political fabric. The emerging welfare state came to rely on the professional practice of welfare professions – their knowledge and discretion. In the early formation of the welfare state, welfare professions were given a central role in the formulation, development and implementation of welfare policies. The use of professional power was made central to the governing of the modern welfare state (Wrede, 2001; Evertsson, 2002).

Today the situation is somewhat different. Social and caring welfare professions are still central to governing the welfare state and pivotal in providing welfare services to citizens, but the relationship with the state has changed. During recent decades welfare professions have experienced increased attempts by the welfare state to manage and control their professional practice. The welfare state is still very dependent on professions, but does not fully rely on their professional discretion.

To give a full historical account of the political, social and economic factors behind this change is beyond the scope of this chapter. However, a bird's-eye view on this change seems to indicate that one important factor was the increasing economic cost of developing and providing welfare services. Many welfare states started to look for more rational and efficient ways of producing welfare. And many were the welfare states that after the 1980s followed in the footsteps of the UK and turned to *New Public Management* (NPM). Seen from a perspective of NPM, professional management and discretion does not represent the most rational or effective way to produce welfare services. NPM turned public administrators into public managers, which changed the balance of power in welfare service organisations (Hood, 1995; McLaughlin et al, 2002). Many social and caring welfare professions found that some aspects of their discretion were transferred into the hands of public managers (Tummers et al, 2009; Hangartner and Svaton, 2013). In welfare professions like medicine, social work and nursing, the changing force of NPM was further underpinned by the introduction of *evidence-based practice* (EBP) at the end of the 1990s (Sackett et al, 1996; Roberts and Yeager, 2006).

Opinions on how EBP affects social and caring welfare professions' professional practice have, to put it mildly, gone in different directions among professionals, researchers and policymakers. Some claim that there has been an improvement in that welfare professionals' work now is more evidence-based and effective, others argue that it has not made much of a difference, while others still argue that EBP has created problems (Mullen et al, 2007; Lilienfeld et al, 2013; Avby et al, 2015). There are also considerable differences between different professional groups. For example, the impact of EBP seems to be greater in medicine than in social work (Rexvid et al, 2012). One reason is probably that it is less difficult to develop standardised interventions matching specific problems in medicine than in social work, which deals with a more 'fuzzy' social reality.

In the wake of NPM and EBP, welfare states have started to act as producers of professional knowledge and promoters of professional standards and guidelines (see Chapter Fourteen). Welfare states actively demand that social and caring welfare professions take a responsive stance towards evidence-based practices and that they adapt their professional practice to fit the managerial principles underpinning NPM. Seen from the perspective of the welfare professions, this is a challenge. It is a delicate matter to navigate between the demand to adjust professional practice towards NPM and EBP, and at the same time stay true to, and to exercise, the core values of professional practice – professional autonomy and discretion (see Chapters Five and Thirteen). Traditionally, the legitimacy and social status of professions and their work rest on the use of scientifically produced and academically transferred knowledge; however, in the new welfare political landscape that is emerging around Europe this picture may have to be revised.

Given today's situation, it is not far-fetched to imagine a future where those welfare social and caring professions that are ready to trade in some of their autonomy and discretion are going to be better off in their relationships with the welfare state. If that happens, a new understanding of the concept of 'profession' is under way – a concept where compliance might play the same role for our understanding of 'profession' as autonomy and discretion once did.

The introduction of NPM and EBP is, however, not the only factor in recent history affecting the professional practice of social and caring welfare professions. As described in this book, we are witnessing a change as established welfare policy areas are in a flux. Today, there seems to be a trend among welfare states to merge and reshape welfare services and organisations that have historically been separated. One way to understand these attempts to create new welfare services and organisations is to view them as the emergence of 'new' medical or social problems, or the development of new political perspectives on existing problems. A good illustration of this is the attempts being made to merge organisations and professions within social services and labour market services (see Chapter Sixteen).

Seen from the perspective of the social and caring welfare professions, the merging of policy areas that have historically been separated poses a threat to professional identity and jurisdiction. Welfare professions that once were just neighbours, residing in separate welfare organisations and working with their own clients in accordance with their own ethical guidelines, knowledge base and practices, are now set to negotiate a common ground for professional practice. Interprofessional work that previously took place in the form of inter-organisational cooperation, is now being reshaped as intra-organisational cooperation. If this intraprofessional negotiation goes wrong, there is no safe haven to retreat to. Given the potential threat to professional identity and jurisdiction, it is understandable if welfare professions regard this emergence of new multi-professional organisations with some degree of scepticism. This boundary work over jurisdictional control may well turn out to be a peaceful process of 'give and take', but it might as well be a process where one profession gains in power and status at the expense of another. The outcome of professional boundary work is hard to predict.

Welfare professions' identity in transition

Some of the contributions (for example Chapters Two to Four) deal with the issue of professional identity and how it is shaped by education, work and various conditions for professional practice. Traditional studies of professional identity usually focus on well-established professions, where an assumption is that the forming of professional identity starts during a long training that leads to the right to exercise a certain profession. Among the contributions in this book, we have, however, identified other aspects concerning identity worth highlighting that previous research has not paid much attention to.

Little or no notice has previously been given to what we would like to denominate 'ad hoc-professions', which could tentatively be defined as professions created to satisfy the needs of a particular kind of labour power. The formation of family assistants in Poland (Chapter Ten) is an example of an ad hoc-profession. In this case, family assistants have to coexist with social workers, who have a relatively clear professional identity and a vision of how the profession's future should look. A number of questions can be raised in connection to the situation of the family assistants, and similar ad hoc-professions. Do they have a professional identity? Is it possible for them to develop a professional identity? Will they become anything other than a profession whose only common attribute is a responsibility and client group determined by the state? In the light of this case, and against a background of what seems to be an increased state control of welfare professions, it is possible to imagine the creation of further ad hoc-professions, where the development of professional identity is unclear.

Another aspect that seems to affect welfare professionals' identity is that several independent professions, as a result of welfare states' new organisational solutions, will work together under the 'same roof'. Put another way, they are collocated in the same organisation, work with the same clients and sometimes perform almost the same work tasks. The employment policy reform in Denmark (Chapter Sixteen) is an example of this sort of development. In this case, different professions have been forced into – partly reluctantly – very close collaboration. They no longer have 'their own' clients, since each client at the same time is other profession's client. In other words, the professional jurisdiction has to be shared with others. The question is how welfare professions respond to this kind of situation. The example from Denmark show that social workers in the service centres try to maintain their exclusivity, and they argue that their unique skills are needed in these organisations. On the other hand, it is possible to challenge such a statement. Are the skills and expertise of social workers more unique than the skills of other professionals in these service centres, such as advisers or specialists in social insurance? The main question here is whether collocated professions, that is, those working under the same roof, will remain separated, at least in their self-perception and identity. Or will this way of organising welfare create new professions, for example public welfare workers with multiple expertise and well-developed skills to meet clients and their needs? And how will it then affect professional identity?

Besides the two aspects of professional identity discussed so far and concerning direct state influence, there is a third where the effects of state influence are more indirect. This concerns the gradual transition whereby *occupational professionalism* is challenged by *organisational professionalism* (Evetts, 2009, 2011), affecting welfare professions in several respects (see Chapters Six and Fourteen). In modern theories on professions and professionalism there is an unspoken assumption that a profession is a necessary precondition for professionalism. The idea is that a profession understood as an occupation must be in place for its members to develop professional values.

According to Evetts, one could, until recently, consider an occupation's professionalism as occupational values. Such values include: practitioners' control over the work system such as procedures and priorities; a discourse of professionalism and a code of ethics provided primarily by a professional association alongside sanctions in cases of professional incompetence; collegial authority; a lengthy period of reasonably uniform education followed by training and/or an apprenticeship; and the development of occupational identities, work cultures and so on (Evetts, 2011). However, organisational changes, not least through NPM, which is initiated or encouraged by the state, has forced traditional occupational professionalism to coexist with organisational professionalism. This type of professionalism is primarily focused on the management and control of the organisations professionals are employed in. One reason for this is that social and caring welfare professionals increasingly work in large-scale organisations such as social services, hospitals and schools that are supposed to adhere to the principles of NPM. Traditional professional values (that is, occupational professionalism) are therefore challenged by organisational values of governance, management, external regulation, audit, work standardisation, performance indicators and so on.

Overall, several contributions in this book suggest that the traditional image of social and caring welfare professions' identity may change, partly through the creation of ad-hoc professions and partly by collocating different established professions under the 'same roof'. However, welfare professions' identity might also change as a consequence of the influence of organisational professionalism. In all these cases, this happens through some sort of state involvement.

Whether this is a problem or not is an open question. But since there are signs that state control of welfare professions and their work is increasing, welfare professions' changing identity will probably be a central issue for researchers and the professions themselves for the years to come.

Struggle, conflict and collaboration

Several chapters in the book touch on professional struggles, conflict and competition (see, for example, Chapters Nine and Eleven). This is by no means surprising since much research show that conflict and competition are part of professionals' 'everyday life'. Some researchers would argue that conflict and competition lies at the very heart of the theoretical understanding of 'profession', since professions compete and make claims on jurisdictional control in conflict with other profession (Freidson, 1970a, 1970b; Larson, 1977; Collins, 1979; Parkin, 1979; Murphy, 1984). In the attempts to establish control and to monopolise segments of the labour market, conflicts are more or less unavoidable.

Research on conflicts and competition has typically focused on the interprofessional aspects of professions in dispute, that is, conflicts involving two or more professions in disputes over jurisdiction. A good example of interprofessional struggle over jurisdiction is to be found in Chapter Nine, which discusses the case of physiotherapy in Norway. However, studying social and caring welfare professions makes it clear that struggle and conflict are not limited to interprofessional disputes. Several chapters in this book (such as Chapters Seven and Ten) paint a picture of conflict and struggle between social and caring welfare professions and the welfare state. Seen from a theoretical point of view, conflicts between the welfare state and welfare professions are quite different from interprofessional conflicts. Welfare professions are to a large extent dependent on resources that are managed by the welfare state and imbedded in welfare policies (Evertsson, 2000, 2005; Wrede, 2001).

The jurisdiction of social and caring welfare professionals is conditioned by welfare policy since it is hard, almost impossible, for welfare professions to develop their jurisdiction and to deliver services that are not in line with existing policies. The welfare state is often the main employer of social and caring welfare professionals, and in many European countries the education and training of social and caring welfare professionals are tied to an educational system that is financed by the state. This dependency makes it hard for welfare professions to take full advantage of what is usually considered to be professions' main resource – scientific knowledge (Larson, 1977; Parkin, 1979; Murphy, 1984; Freidson, 1986). The restricted range of scientific knowledge is well illustrated in Chapter Ten on the professional development of social work in Poland after 1989, when the Polish welfare state acted indifferently towards social workers' argument that they were the best qualified professionals to work with individuals and families with complex needs. In this specific case it seems like staffing – in the sense of finding enough manpower – was a more pressing issue than best professional competence. The possibility for welfare professions to use scientific knowledge as a strategic resource may also be restricted by current trends for welfare states to act as producers of knowledge and promoters of professional standards and guidelines in the name of NPM and EBP.

Another theme in the book is professional collaboration. Welfare professions have always had to collaborate with each other, but seen from a historical perspective the forms for professional collaboration have changed. Whereas early forms of collaboration between welfare professions often took the shape of serial processing of clients between welfare professions residing in different organisations, collaboration today tends to build on multi-professional teams or organisations. As the chapters in this book indicate (for example, Chapters Eight, Twelve and Sixteen), these forms of multi-professional collaboration do not always work in the intended way, since they involve negotiation of different jurisdictional claims, coordination of different professional competences and practices, and the merging of different ethical values. Hence, welfare professional collaboration in multi-professional settings involves boundary work.

Against this background, it is important to recognise that the presence of collaboration does not mean the absence of conflict; on the contrary, it is likely that collaboration in some cases stirs up conflict. However, taking one of the biggest challenges facing social and caring welfare professions, namely how to gain bargaining strength to influence welfare policymaking, multi-professional settings could provide a platform for new professional alliances. Yet, for this to occur welfare, professions might need to play down the professional identity politics that many welfare professions of today pursue. The quest for a refined and unique professional identity that supports the jurisdictional claims being made can very well prove to be one of the biggest problems of establishing collaboration between welfare professions.

Knowledge as a tool in direct practice or a means for controlling professionals?

The tension between professional discretion and managerial control is sometimes described as a conflict between occupational professionalism and organisational professionalism (Evetts, 2011). Seen from the perspective of the welfare state and its welfare organisations, managerial control is closely related to issues of service quality, transparency, accountability and optimal use of resources. Seen from the perspective of the welfare professions, increased managerial control is interpreted as distrust. More problematic, however, is that the increased level of managerial control is perceived as a loss of professional discretion and the core elements of professional practice get lost or go unnoticed.

As noted in several of the chapters (for example, Chapters Thirteen to Fifteen), professional practice – screening, assessments, decision making and intervention – is far from an instrumental use of knowledge. On the contrary, professional practice is also creative work. However, these non-instrumental aspects of professional practice tend to go unnoticed in a managerial world where professional practice is seen as a linear and instrumental process.

The tension between occupational professionalism and organisational professionalism has made professional knowledge the centre of attention. Professional knowledge is becoming the new battlefield where the welfare state and the welfare professions play out their differences. Today we are witnessing a situation where the welfare state takes on a new role as producer and promoter of professional knowledge. The knowledge promoted often has a 'hands-on' character, involving manuals, guidelines, protocols and standardised instruments for screening, assessments and interventions. But there is also a new situation for professions of the welfare state since jurisdictional claims must be sensitive towards knowledge promoted by the welfare state.

Seen from the perspective of the social and caring welfare professions, it can be a tightrope act to establish a professional practice that stays 'true' to the fundamental perspectives and core values of the profession, and at the same time is sensitive towards the guidelines, protocols, manuals and standardised instruments for screening, assessment and intervention promoted by the welfare state. This task becomes even more daunting in the wake of the development of new policy areas, such as employment-oriented social work, where established professional jurisdictions are questioned, as different welfare professions set out to work together closely. The current trend towards managerial control shows little sign of decreasing, which leaves advocates of occupational professionalism with little hope (see Chapter Five).

However, in Denmark and Sweden, initiatives have been taken indicating that there are ambitions to increase social and caring welfare professions' opportunities to govern themselves. What makes this particularly interesting is that these initiatives have been launched by the national governments. In 2013, the Danish government and the parties in the public sector made an agreement, the so-called 'trust reform' (*Tillidsreform*), which is a counter-reaction to New Public Management. According to Danish researchers (Pedersen and Tangkjær, 2013; Thygesen and Kampmann, 2013), the principles behind NPM, including different types of management and control, were applied to such an extent that they have become counter-productive, and have created mistrust between actors in the welfare sector. The 'trust reform' involves creating management systems in the public sector, based less on control and more on responsibility and trust in employees' professionalism and ability to lead themselves. The Swedish government has taken similar steps, by initiating a process of developing new models of public management that would give professional ethics and discretion a more prominent position within public services (Swedish Government, 2014-2015). Whether these examples are just single events in two Scandinavian countries or signs of a broader trend is still an open question.

Conclusion

The future is always around the corner and it is hard to know what it entails. This chapter has touched on some key issues that highlight the conditions for the social and caring welfare professions in different European welfare states. As the book shows, social and caring welfare professions exist in many different guises, which, of course, reflects peoples' varying needs and problems. It is also a result of various welfare systems in different countries. However, at the same time there is something common and unifying in the multifaceted, since social and caring welfare professions aim to maintain or improve people's lives on behalf of the public. This common trait runs like a thread through the various contributions, and we believe that the book is therefore also relevant to professions and countries that are not explicitly discussed.

One ambition of this book is to offer research-based knowledge on various aspects of social and caring welfare professions in a European perspective. It is probably safe to assume that welfare professions will continue to exist, evolve and increase, both in Europe and other parts of the world for the foreseeable future, not least against the background of rapid economic and social development in many Asian, African and South American countries, which can lead to a changing relationship between state, professions and citizens. Which welfare professions will exist in the future, and what challenges they will face, are hard to predict and will be questions for future research. We have tried to contribute with insights about contemporary social and caring welfare professions that may benefit those who set the terms for professions, as well as professions themselves. By offering decision makers, professionals and students new understandings, we hope that those who are in need of welfare services – clients, patients, users, and so on – will receive help better suited to maintaining or improving their welfare and wellbeing.

References

Avby, G., Nilsen, P. and Ellström, P.E. (2015) 'Exploring evidence-based practice in practice – the case of social work', in M. Elg, P.-E. Ellström, M. Klofsten and M. Tillmar (eds) *Sustainable development in organizations: Studies on innovative practices*, Cheltenham: Edward Elgar Publishing, pp 153-68.

Collins, R. (1979) *The credential society. A historical sociology of education and stratification*, New York, NY: Academic Press.

Evertsson, L. (2000) 'The Swedish welfare state and the emergence of female welfare state occupations', *Gender, Work and Organization*, 7(4): 230-41.

Evertsson, L. (2002) *Välfärdspolitik och kvinnoyrken. Organisation, välfärdsstat och professionaliseringens villkor* [Welfare policy and female-dominated occupations. Organisation, welfare state and conditions for professionalization], Umeå: Umeå Universitet, Sociologiska Institutionen.

Evetts, J. (2009) 'New professionalism and new public management: changes, continuities and consequences', *Comparative Sociology*, 8(2): 247-66.

Evetts, J. (2011) 'A new professionalism? Challenges and opportunities', *Current Sociology*, 59(4): 406-22.

Freidson, E. (1970a) *Professional dominance: The social structure of medicial care*, New York, NY: Atherton Press.

Freidson, E. (1970b) *Profession of medicine: A study of the sociology of applied knowledge*, New York, NY: Harper & Row.

Freidson, E. (1986) *Professional powers*, Chicago, IL: University of Chicago Press.

Hangartner, J. and Svaton, C.J. (2013) 'From autonomy to quality management: NPM impacts on school governance in Switzerland', *Journal of Educational Administration and History*, 45(4): 354-69.

Hood, C. (1995) 'The "New Public Management" in the 1980s: variations on a theme', *Accounting, Organizations and Society*, 20(2): 93-109.

Larson, S.M. (1977) *The rise of professionalism. A sociological analysis*, Berkeley, CA: Berkeley University Press.

Lilienfeld, S.O., Ritschel, L.A., Lynn, S.J., Cautin, R.L. and Latzman, R.D. (2013) 'Why many clinical psychologists are resistant to evidence-based practice: root causes and constructive remedies', *Clinical Psychology Review*, 33(7): 883-900.

McLaughlin, K., Osborne, S.P. and Ferlie, E. (eds) (2002) *New Public Management: Current trends and future prospects*, London and New York, NY: Routledge.

Mullen, E.J., Bledsoe, S.E. and Bellamy, J. L. (2008) 'Implementing evidence-based social work practice', *Research on Social Work Practice*, 8(4): 325-38

Murphy, R. (1984) 'The structure of closure: a critique and development of Weber, Collins and Parkin', *British Journal of Sociology*, 35(4): 547-67.

Parkin, F. (1979) *Marxism and class theory. A bourgeois critique*, London: Tavistock Publications.

Pedersen, D. and Tangkjær, C. (2013) 'Building leadership capacity in the involving network state', *Teaching Public Administration*, 31(1): 29-41.

Rexvid, D., Blom, B., Evertsson, L. and Forssén, A. (2012) 'Risk reduction technologies in general practice and social work', *Professions and Professionalism*, 2(2): 1-18.

Roberts, A.R. and Yeager, K. (2006) *Foundations of evidence-based social work practice*, New York, NY: Oxford University Press.

Sackett, D.L., Rosenberg, W.M., Gray, J.M., Haynes, R.B. and Richardson, W.S. (1996) 'Evidence based medicine: what it is and what it isn't', *British Medical Journal*, 312(7023): 71-2.

Swedish Government (2014-2015) 'Ny styrning bortom New Public Management' [New governance beyond the New Public Management], Press release, first published 23 October 2014, updated 2 April 2015, www.regeringen.se/pressmeddelanden/2014/10/ny-styrning-bortom-new-public-management.

Thygesen, N. and Kampmann, N.E.S. (2013) *Tillid på bundlinjen: Offentlige ledere går nye veje* [Confidence on the bottom line: Public managers are breaking new ground], Copenhagen: Gyldendal.

Tummers, L., Bekkers, V. and Steijn, B. (2009) 'Policy alienation of public professionals: application in a New Public Management context', *Public Management Review*, 11(5): 685-706.

Wrede, S. (2001) *Decentering care for mothers. The politics of midwifery and the design of Finnish maternity services*, Åbo: Åbo Akademi University Press.

Index

T

U

V

W

Y

Lightning Source UK Ltd.
Milton Keynes UK
UKHW020058100819
347744UK00008B/572/P